Poverty
~
Hunger
~
Disease
~
and Global Health

Don A. Franco

Published by Yawn's Publishing
210 East Main Street
Canton, GA 30114
www.yawnsbooks.com

This book is printed exactly as the author intended, without editorial input or reference verification from Yawn's Publishing.

ISBN 978-0-9796231-0-3

Printed in the United States of America.

Photo credits – Pages iii and 32 (S. Foster), 81, 88, 193 (C. Zahniser), 200 (J. Noble Jr), 217, and 223 – Centers for Disease Control and Prevention; Pages xii, 51, and 181 (M. Uz Zaman) – Food and Agriculture Organization of the United Nations; Pages 24, 56 (A. Fiorente), 66, 133 (D. Budd-Gray), 142, 152 (Y. Abo Gadr), 170, 213, and 227 – World Health Organization; Pages 106, 109, and 121 – Nobelprize.org.

Acknowledgements

The subject of poverty and the domino effect of it on society, especially in the developing countries, must be addressed with urgency, if not immediacy. This, my latest book, Poverty, Hunger, Disease and Global Health, is a small token to the many dedicated people who are sincerely intent and motivated to make the world a better place for all by committing their time, talent, and resources with the hope of creating change and new vistas for the world's 3 billion forgotten people dreaming of better tomorrows.

I give special thanks to family and many friends who share my vision. I pay homage to James (Jim) Andreoli of the Jerome Foundation (Los Angeles) for his encouragement, support, and friendship. Jim shares the same dreams by reaching out to various uplifting programs in the Philippines to make life and living a little better. As a global society, we must all suppress the indignities of poverty and create reasons for optimism. We owe it to humanism.

Tina Caparella, a friend of many years, continues to "play" with my manuscripts, and her "games" have always contributed to improvements that I could not envision myself. I express, once more, my utmost appreciation to Tina for bringing the book to closure.

Foreword

I have written *Poverty, Hunger, Disease and Global Health* to addend my two previous publication attempts to address the inequalities caused by global poverty and its impact on hunger, disease, and social justice. This effort was completed during a passage of my life, at age 79, when most of our age have given up on the greater game of involvement and caring that could contribute to positive solutions for a better world. We still have numerous pressing challenges to overcome throughout the globe, including the continuing existence of a global health crisis linked to poverty.

Humanism dictates that we must prevail in our quest to alleviate the blight and suffering caused by widespread poverty. Success in our efforts will make the world a better and more livable experience for billions who continue to live with little hope of better tomorrows.

"Is there some meaning to this life? What purpose lies behind the strife?
Whence do we come, where are we bound?
These cold questions echo and resound through each day,
    each lonely night.
We long to find the splendid night that will cast a revelatory beam
    upon the meaning of the human dream."
The Book of Counted Sorrows

Contents

Preface

The only objective of writing a book that relates to poverty, hunger, and disease applicable to global health, with mostly depressing themes, amplified by uncertainty and discouraging evidence, is to indulge in reasoned discourse and informed scrutiny of the subject. Additionally, it is a concerted effort to contribute to the debate by highlighting poverty as the causal "domino" of hunger and disease, during a period when the global public health community continues to examine new options and goals to alleviate poverty and modify or help change the current inequities and inequalities that exist throughout the world.

The book's introduction provides a general overview of the nuances of poverty, hunger, and disease globally, and the contradictory impasse that shows evidence of progress and success in some regions of the world, mixed with signs of hopelessness and despair in others, and an obvious mandate for a new agenda for the future because of the challenging disparities.

Chapters 1 and 2 review the historical record by analyzing the philosophical intent of the Universal Declaration of Human Rights, and the United Nations/World Health Organization "Health for All by the Year 2000" objectives by debating and questioning the hyper-inflated and haughty language of these two major declarations while by-passing the varying dimensions of reality when establishing responses and proposing policies that will affect health and well-being of people globally.

Chapter 3 assesses the all-embracing Millennium Development Goals (MDGs) by detailing each of the eight established goals and subjecting each to reasoned evaluations within the projected timeframe for likely achievement. The discussion begs the question whether or not many of the goals could not have been considered with more restraint, regardless of their utmost worthiness, which were meant to address the acuteness of the existing wrongs globally.

Chapters 4, 5, and 6 analyze the fundamental affronts to public health in predominantly developing countries by examining the

i

association and cumulative problems of water, sanitation and hygiene, the history and constant burden of infectious diseases, and the new dimensions of chronic diseases that have started to overwhelm the resources and global public health infrastructure of all countries, but, especially, the severe negative impact of these diseases on emerging economies.

Chapter 7 and 8 were developed to examine the linkages of hunger and malnutrition to health in resource-poor countries and the concomitant widespread inequities between the developed and the developing countries, while proposing an agenda for the consideration of sustainable food production as a logical option, bordering on imperative, for improving the health of people in underdeveloped societies in a world still fraught with blatant inequalities.

Chapters 9 and 10 delved into a mixture of both retrospective and futuristic aspects of global health challenges by examining the broad and continuing impasse of the health and disease status of populations in the mostly developing world, and whether or not there is any evidence that would heighten now or in the foreseeable future hope and optimism in a world of distinct uncertainties.

The epilogue epitomized the past with the acceptance that change was needed, and hope and optimism could only be fully accomplished with a more realistic and balanced agenda for the future. The traditional hyper-inflation of goals, regardless of how worthy they may be, will never guarantee progress or success. In fact, they could serve as deterrents and demoralizing. Results will be dependent on the commitment and proper use of the collective resources of individual countries with the anticipated long-term support and collaboration of organizations that remain prepared to make life and living a more meaningful experience for the world's less fortunate. A global health crisis exists, and it is linked to poverty. History will ultimately judge how well we do through interventions to benefit global public health, and, in the process, to improve the lot of humanity.

Introduction

Any author's attempt to address the subject of poverty, hunger, and disease and its obvious relationship and connectedness to the major pathologies affecting global health is fraught with soul-searching frustration, uncertainty, disappointment, and doubt. One is often left feeling a continuing sense of concern and trepidation that little can be done that will cause meaningful and measureable change in the poverty alleviation and health status of people worldwide, exemplified by the challenges that the developing countries face and will likely continue to face for many years. This situation continues to discourage and frustrate, even in the midst of some shadows of light and reasons for guarded hope and optimism in the last two decades. The historical record of poverty, hunger, and disease globally remains in the realm of contentious debate at the dawn of the 21st century, forcing all with a genuine and dedicated interest in global health to pursue the search for needed solutions that could contribute to positive change in the future. Each theme has varying pathologies that have defied the world health community for decades. The variables are reflected in the reactions and opinions of medical/public health professionals who are intent on making correctives that will sustain progress and maintain long-term

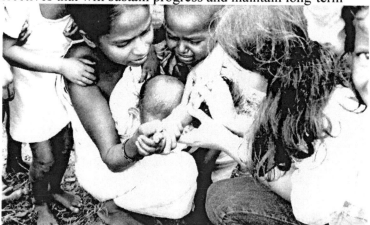

change, especially in the emerging economies.

Many leaders in global health project a sense of optimism, highlighting gains and accomplishments in the last two decades, while others express utter despair paralleling hopelessness, and the opinion that we still have a long road to travel before any positive claims can be made. This obvious contradictory impasse should be anticipated, but it tends to perpetuate a mixture of helplessness, disappointment, and disillusionment, creating a sense of doubt whether global health planners and leaders have any idea where we are or where we plan to go, and, above all, how we hope to get there now, and, in the future. And, obviously, the added concern, who will lead us to the light and the answers that will create the needed changes? That question is not unreasonable in the fractious and disorganized world of global health with all the disparate programs with far-reaching objectives that appear lacking in direction, mission, unification, and vision, in spite of the most noble and well-meant intentions of the myriad organizations and dedicated people working to ensure change. In fact, that and similar type questions have plagued the global health landscape for decades, particularly in regions where progress has been marginal to non-existent. This challenging dilemma can become an opportunity for reexamination and a renewed sense of purpose that can foster policy modifications, and a new direction with opportunities for sustained change. In essence, regardless of what side of the debate you are on and how contentious and impossible the issues seem, we of the global health community still have a long and tortuous road to travel based on the historical record and the uncertain future of the world order.

Successful health programs necessitate maintaining both an ongoing communication and collaboration between the providers and recipients of health care services and must include a continuous evaluation of the established objectives, whether at the local, national, or global levels. At the global level, people throughout the world have shown that regardless of their cultural and other differences, they strive for an improved standard of living and the hope for a life of dignity and happiness, including the embrace of ready access to equitable health care when available and needed. But, any change or transformation of health policies and care globally involves the continuing variables and complex subject of managing the disease risks that people are subjected to. Realistically, only those countries that have the resources and the infrastructure to respond and do something truly contributory to engender change will have any hope to achieve their goals.

Indeed, the World Health Organization's (WHO's) "Health for all 2000" deserves reasoned debate and criticism for the outcome deficits. But, at least, people assembled to do something at Alma-Ata in 1978, about correcting the plight of global health, so credit is due the visionaries who assembled to correct the wrongs of the past and establish goals for the future. You may not want to celebrate what they hoped to accomplish and did not, but, they acted in good faith. Additionally, particularly in the case of global health care, our continuing primary concern, success can be improved and enhanced if people could start considering themselves global citizens, and work within the philosophical objective that we are all in this together. This is one of those utopian suggestions that continue to emerge in objectifying the attributes of global health during the past three decades. But, it never seems to be fully embraced outside the world of the medical and public health globalists who are truly convinced that the concept of a global citizen is applicable for long-term progressivism to advance a holistic health agenda for the vulnerable poor throughout the world.

Using hypothetical examples to make the point of global togetherness, the German public health specialist in tropical medicine communicating with colleagues in Guatemala City must have that ingrained empathy and understanding of the unique problems of a country like Guatemala, or any other developing country for that matter. During the sojourn, he/she or they, must feel and think like a Guatemalan and their anxieties and needs must be foremost in the formatting of objectives for change. Their collaboration must be in unison and mutual respect to benefit the advancement of medical knowledge and public health globally. The same theory applies to the many medical/public health scientists from industrialized countries working in resource-poor settings under trying conditions and at times great personal sacrifices to influence change. Interestingly, so many of the "foreign" professionals working to improve health in developing countries have very humane attributes and never think in terms of the sacrificial perspective, but more toward aspects of how they can make a difference and truly influence change!

At the other end of the spectrum, the Indian, Pakistani, Nigerian, or any other nationality graduate students, studying at medical and public health institutions in the developed and industrialized societies, must embrace the opportunity from both a maximal and optimal point of view and seek alliances that could result in research collaborations for long-term mutual benefits to solve problems of their home countries, while building meaningful professional alliances and friendships with their hosts. They should behave like happy guests swimming in a sea of knowledge with dreams of doing good things for their home countries and the advancement of medicine and public health. This could be a vaccine for malaria or hookworm, the development of an improved medicine to treat drug resistant tuberculosis, or simply working on the development of generic medicines to control and prevent diseases and improve health in their native lands. The ultimate goal remains, and should always be - the bringing together of diverse resources for the collective good to improve people's health throughout the globe. The concept of a global citizen for the advancement of health has definite validity and should be promoted.

The continuing challenges of the varied aspects/concepts and degrees of existing poverty globally are difficult to define precisely and are heightened and complicated by the accompanying residual and domino effect of malnutrition, hunger, disease, and inequality, cumulatively, all of which defy traditional corrective solutions that have been tried in the past and failed, contributing to the current dilemma and differing opinions that continue to cloud the subject and demand an assessment of new vistas. It has now become increasingly obvious that new perspectives are needed to examine currency and determine whether or not a new approach to examine poverty, hunger, and the entirety of global health/disease prevention goals is not an absolute if we have any hope of addressing and correcting the present and future realm and direction of poverty alleviation in all its negative dimensions throughout the world, and the concurrent impact that poverty, in general, has on populations most at risk in developing societies.

It is impossible to separate hunger and disease from poverty. They are completely interrelated and pertinently connected, contributing to a challenging social and public health dilemma for decision-makers and planners in all of the middle and low income countries of the world. This circumstantial condition perpetuates a feeling of despair and helplessness, and the acceptance that a global health crisis exists, and it is directly associated with global poverty. The thought that a low of 800 million to more than a billion people go without enough food every day in a world of unparalleled wealth, where plenty of food is available, becomes a compelling challenge for all leaders and policy makers in the global fight to eliminate the blight of poverty. And, for the first time in the history of world hunger statistics, one sixth of humanity or over 1.02 billion people do not have enough to eat (exceeding the combined population of the United States, Canada, and the European Union). Equally disconcerting is in this milieu at least 16,000 young lives are lost to the indignity of hunger every day, in a world of abundance.

The disturbing finding that more than half of the world's population, or over three billion people, fit into the poor category, and over one billion are considered extremely poor, amplifies the depressing dilemma and mandates an imperative for renewed prioritized action and the introduction and consideration of new initiatives and goals if we have any hope to promote semblances of health equity and justice for the poorest of the poor on our planet. Common decency dictates that we must act now, and above all, must not fail. It should be thought of as a priority humanitarian concern and resolve, because the ravages and blight of poverty continue to prevent poor countries from providing the resources and leadership needed to prevent malnutrition, hunger and control diseases, and the needed opportunities for promoting improved health, and, hopefully, economic welfare in the future. The fact is that 18 million people die annually from poverty-related causes or approximately 50,000 deaths daily. These numbers coming from WHO are without doubt a conservative estimate at best. The report, however, should amplify concerns that immediacy must become the response factor to address the existing inequities that afflict the poor globally if we have any hope of creating an environment for meaningful progressivism and change.

I cannot help but reflect on the draconian efforts of the Irish born rock star, Bono, and his totality of social awareness as he looked at the eyes of the hungry of Africa as sensitized in the lyrics of the Beatles, "Imagine all the people." His equally passionate lobbying of the British Parliament and the United States Congress on behalf of the poor has become an education in morality and an exemplar for emulation to show that individual actions could be a source of power to change attitudes and help in the creation of an agenda for the elimination of poverty in a world that flourishes with plenty. His ability to make former Senator Jesse Helms of North Carolina, an icon of Republican conservatism, listen to his pleas and consider the entirety of the problems linked to poverty and the resulting negative impact on millions of people throughout the globe is a study in persuasion. The senator's historical attitude towards foreign aid to developing countries has been one of waste triggered by corruption and poor governance and no accountability by recipients. That was by no means an unreasonable reaction of the senator based on investigative findings over the years. Bono, nonetheless, persisted with patience and pleas for the senator to consider the pressing and compelling basic needs of the poor globally. He ultimately developed an excellent working relationship with the senator based on an evolving mutual respect. This alliance of two people with strong opinions and distinctly different political persuasions resulted in benefits through increased funding for many of the world's most destitute people!

Unfortunately, individualism, even of the dynamism of a personality like Bono could be enhanced by fate and destiny. That occurred eventually, and brought the commitment and dreams of the superstar in definite commonality with the mission/vision of the Bill and Melinda Gates Foundation, the largest foundation in the world. This coming together of the two resources started the evolution of a broad and comprehensive set of progressive programs to address some of the urgent needs of the poor globally. This beneficial togetherness of Bono and the Gates Foundation culminated in their contributions being recognized as Time's Persons of the Year in 2006: "For being shrewd about doing good, for rewriting politics and reengineering justice, for making mercy smarter and hope strategic and the daring the rest of us to follow."

While Bono continues with the same love and commitment to the cause of the underprivileged poor, the Bill and Melinda Gates Foundation has become the most influencing force in global health by targeting huge monetary support for control of diseases in the developing countries, especially highlighting malaria, HIV/AIDS, and tuberculosis. The accompanying philosophical mantra of the foundation is that all lives have equal value, whether it is a destitute child in an African shack or an offspring of the super-rich in Europe or America. This mantra for doing good has spread like an epidemic and known celebrities and several organizations have joined to play significant roles in the cause of poverty elimination, or, at least, contributing to development and a better standard of living for the poor in developing countries.

Additionally, the Gates Foundation supports research and institutions throughout the world that will improve and contribute to solutions that are practical, affordable, and effective to help the general health conditions of people, especially those incapable of helping themselves, the poor and vulnerable. The visionaries of the Bill and Melinda Gates Foundation are conscious that the alleviation of poverty, health promotion, and disease control in the less developed countries of the world, exemplified by sub-Saharan Africa, and parts of Asia and Latin America, cannot be accomplished without investments in agriculture and food production. The future direction and thought was that hunger could one day become marginalized in many developing countries if national governments made food production a top priority and embrace in the process the emerging technologies in agriculture to boost food production to self-sufficiency, and, hopefully, evolve into a surplus one day.

The underlying objective and potential of this futuristic perspective in agricultural policy was to examine a "green" approach as integral to the process of improvement, and heighten crop production in a responsible way while conforming to the customary farming practices and traditions of the people, and optimizing the acquired know-how from emerging technology in genetics and land use to maximum advantage. This, it was thought, could only be achieved by working in coalition with the farmers themselves and respecting their inputs and advice and planning in unison through active participation. In essence, the goal simply was that we are all in this together as equals, no dictating from a donor organization, and follow what you are told approach as was so customary. Empowerment of people in the farming community and active collaboration with technical support staff and agricultural specialists became the operational theme. That would hopefully result one day in feeding millions of people on the African continent and other developing countries, saving lives, and ultimately reducing the burden of poverty, improving the standard of living, and providing a reason for hope in a region that has historically not celebrated the beauty and blessings of hope.

While the work done by Bono and the Gates Foundation receive a lot of media attention because of the personalities involved, a lot of other organizations are having a positive influence on change throughout the globe. The Carter Center in partnership with Emory University (my alma mater), has as its major objective and commitment the advancement of human rights, the alleviation of unnecessary human suffering, and the creation of a world in which every man, woman, and child has the opportunity to enjoy good health and live in peace. The Center's vision conforms to the heart of the Universal Declaration of Human Rights that will be discussed in the next chapter.

Doctors Without Borders (Medicins Sans Frontieres) is an international medical organization that is private and not-for-profit whose main function is humanitarian in scope. The organization has 19 national branches throughout the world with an international office in Geneva, Switzerland. The organization functions in concert with its name – a well-defined mission and vision to enhance global humanitarianism especially in medical relief supplies and health related research activities in treatment of the sick and poor.

The Clinton Global Initiative (CGI) functions under the auspices of the William J. Clinton Foundation that highlights the benefits of the integration of a global community of responsibilities and values hoping to serve as a catalyst for change by bringing world leaders together to study and apply innovative solutions to some of the world's most challenging problems. CGI's glo0bal periscope focuses on poverty alleviation, global health with emphasis on the broad realm of disease control with emphasis on HIV/AIDS, the control of tropical diseases, and the promotion of global public health initiatives.

There is always a danger in identifying the multiplicity of organizations involved for any reason. The tendency is to leave out one or another, person or organization, doing excellent service and cause offense. Obviously, I seek understanding that all those doing good for humanity, many without transparency, could not be included, and I beg forgiveness. But, mention must be made of the many private donors who readily come to mind and have contributed so much to the betterment of life for so many throughout the world. Many global initiatives that benefit the poor of the world would never have been completed without the generosity of organizations like the Rockefeller Foundation, the MacArthur Foundation, the Kellogg Foundation, the Edna McConnell Clark Foundation, the Kaiser Family Foundation, the Turner Foundation, Oxfam, the

Howard Hughes Medical Institute, Save the Children, Catholic Relief, and Rotary Foundation. To these organizations and all who have given so much – the cause of humanity has benefited through their unselfish outreach. Granted that a listing of this nature could never be truly all inclusive, we pay homage, nonetheless, to all who have in small or grandiose ways influenced the lives and living conditions of so many in dire need throughout the world.

A cloud of darkness, however, still surrounds us globally. About 30,000 children still die each day throughout the world before they reach the age of five because of the varying poor living conditions and environmental degradation that contribute to different stages of morbidity and sickness that often culminates in death, affirming the powerful influence of the pathology of poverty under which the majority of people living in developing countries still face daily. Fifty percent of the world's children still live in poverty, and over six hundred million live in primitive conditions devoid of any form of shelter or security.

About half a billion children worldwide still lack access to clean water. More alarming is that dirty water and poor sanitation are responsible for the majority of the 1.8 million child deaths from different forms of diarrhea, or about 5,000 deaths daily, making diarrhea as a global disease complex the second largest cause of child mortality. Sadly, deaths from diarrhea are preventable with oral rehydration salts that are comparatively cheap and effective if properly used. Additionally, of the 2.2 billion children in the world, 600 million are victims of extreme poverty. This is doubtless a conservative estimate when the populations at risk are fully assessed and evaluated from a global perspective. Nonetheless,

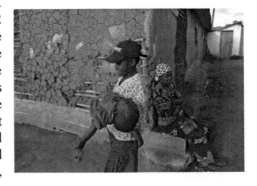

the statistical evidence is overwhelming and illuminates the acuteness of the global affront of poverty as a risk factor and the corrective mandates needed.

The current global economic slowdown has expectedly become a challenge and the Food and Agriculture Organization (FAO) has projected that about 100 million more people will enter the depressing world of poverty and hunger by the end of 2009, about an 11% increase over 2008. Even in an affluent society like the United States, for comparative reference, more than 33 million people including 13 million children live in households that are at risk of hunger or experience hunger. According to the World Bank about 1.4 billion people suffer from extreme poverty or trying to live on the purchasing power of $1.25 (U.S.) daily, mostly living in regions of the world with poor governance, fragile institutions, and burdened by war, refugee camps, political terrorism, and malnutrition/hunger and disease. Countries of sub-Saharan Africa typify, unfortunately, all of the major depressing statistics associated with extreme poverty.

Hunger will doubtless persist as a global health risk factor for years and a potential affront to good progressive governance in many developing countries, especially in some of the most destitute countries of the world. It will remain the most apparent symptom of world poverty unless a concerted and collective effort is made by donor countries and institutions and the national governments of the affected countries to institute agricultural policies that would make food production a top priority and turn the tide toward some semblance of meaningful agricultural sustainability that will make food available at a price that people can afford. This consideration to be successful should be pursued with the same intensity as the Marshall Plan embarked on by the United States to assist countries of Western Europe after the Second World War to build their shattered infrastructure and start the economic turnaround in the region. The success of the Marshall Plan is legend and compelling. This type of initiative could be complementary and in concert with what the Gates Foundation has started with agricultural priorities in some countries in Africa and be enhanced by micro-finance as proposed by Muhammad Yunus in the battle against poverty. It would be ludicrous to assume that micro-credit methods that worked in Bangladesh could not have a successful applicability to developing countries in other regions of the globe, including the many countries of sub-Saharan Africa in most need of that type of financing.

Micro-lending could, therefore, be the "stimulus package" to make development work in poor countries by offering people small loans for agricultural or other endeavors like cottage industries toward the hope of self-sufficiency. This objective could be the biggest factor in helping poor people, in resource-poor countries, experience an opportunity for building and improving their own economic plight, while assisting a nation's potential for sustainable economic growth, and, in the process, poverty alleviation. Properly executed we are looking at the possibility of a win-win outcome and optimism for all involved if the principles of micro-finance as practiced by the Grameen Bank are followed with care as was the case with the village people of Bangladesh who showed the world that a bank for the poor could be the new economics for developing countries.

Conversely, while poverty and hunger remains an albatross around our necks, over 270 million people, a very conservative estimate, do not know what it is like to enjoy any access to basic or rudimentary health services. This is so for a multitude of reasons, all predominantly linked to varying aspects of poverty, and the existing social and economic conditions of poor societies. Most people in developing countries cannot afford even some of the basic expenses of medical care and often have to forego seeing doctors for treatment or needed interventions, resulting in negative health consequences, and at times the unfortunate reality of premature death. This begs the obvious question, why in spite of all the promotional hype and thousands of initiatives in the last three decades about the urgency to end poverty and the consequences of it, we are still struggling, albeit, with some signs of definite progress in some sectors, to demonstrate signs of measurable and meaningful progress that we can all truly celebrate? In some sectors of the world, the problem of poverty, hunger, and disease has become progressively worse, mocking our ingenuity, and challenging our resolve.

The global disease profile continues to be a disturbing challenge to those with an interest in diseases of poverty when the three primary diseases of the poor, HIV/AIDS, malaria, and tuberculosis are contextualized. The prevalence of AIDS is 95% in developing countries, and one person is infected with the HIV virus every 6.4 seconds. The percentage for active tuberculosis is a staggering 98% with someone in the world dying of the disease every 18 seconds. Additionally, 90% of malaria deaths occur in sub-Saharan Africa, or about 125 deaths every hour. Cumulatively, these three diseases alone are responsible for 10% of global mortality. These percentages and statistics highlight and amplify the overwhelming burden of infectious diseases in predominantly poor countries worldwide.

Measles, pneumonia, and diarrhea in its different manifestations are also closely associated with poverty. Maternal and neonatal deaths addend the complexity for disease control initiatives in developing countries where 98% of the approximate 12,000 deaths occur daily. This continual cycle of poverty and disease in developing countries, particularly in sub-Saharan Africa contributes to an economic and public health crisis. Finally, the thought that eight million people die every year because they are simply just too destitute to stay alive due to extreme poverty, chronic hunger, lack of minimal health resource or care, and no access to clean drinking water or a sanitary environment illuminate the disease burden.

While infectious diseases remain a compelling and distinct challenge in developing countries, one would be remiss not to consider the impact of the neglected tropical diseases (NTDs) that affect one in every six people on earth. These diseases thrive in areas of extreme poverty in places with unsafe water, poor sanitation, and limited or no access to basic healthcare facilities. Interestingly, most of these diseases can be prevented or eliminated to minimize morbidity and mortality, but since they pose a very limited threat to developed countries, and do not represent a lucrative investment or market for medicines, they remain in the neglected category in the realm of research. An additional affront to global public health is the comparative affordability and simple diagnostic tools needed for some of the NTDs. In spite of this, many people in remote regions of the developing countries become sick and die because the diagnostic regimens require skilled workers to perform them. That support mechanism is in short supply and as often is the case simply not available in most countries. The opportunities for collaborative research with developed countries are endless considering that the joint efforts of all people throughout the world of medicine are what life is all about.

For decades, public health reports and initiatives have advocated that a concerted battle is needed to conquer the indignity and blight of poverty, hunger, disease, ignorance, educational inequities, and indifference. The advent of the twenty-first century has again energized these cries for seeking a path to improve the quality of life of millions of people living in dire need and totally vulnerable. The needs remain so widespread, acute, and complex that a rededication is a mandate. Unless we correct and improve on the depressing problems that exist in the poor countries of the globe, we all become vulnerable and directly exposed to the realities of disease transmission through globalization, travel, and trade.

Public health is an integral component of social justice, and an important element of a country's development. That analogy should provide ample hope for the future and provide a path for us to take and a long-term commitment to make the world a more livable place for the many unfortunate who are presently roaming and feeling lost and hopeless during a period when there ought to be semblances of hope for better tomorrows. Our response to poverty and the concurrent domino effect is so much like doubting schizophrenics – we are unable to understand the irony of it all – the more things change, the more they remain the same!

The intent of the book is to fully examine the nuances of poverty, malnutrition/hunger and the disease perspective globally by starting with the Universal Declaration of Human Rights, and major United Nations' programs like Health for All by the Year 2000, the Millennium Development Goals (MDGs), a re-examination of disease prevalence, both infectious and chronic with special emphasis on developing countries, theories of malnutrition and hunger, and a proposal that sustainable food production could be a major public health resource. The book will finally reiterate the major aspects of the challenges of public health in developing countries while asking the question that the world of public health practice has been asking for nearly a century, Is there reason for optimism?

Our world should be a world that is free of poverty, and I close with a dream for change as written by a dreamer, and stands in the lobby of the World Bank in Washington, D.C.:

> *If we act now with realism and foresight,*
> *If we show courage,*
> *If we think globally and allocate our resources accordingly,*
> *We can give our children a more peaceful and equitable world.*
> *One where suffering will be reduced.*
> *Where children everywhere will have a sense of hope.*
> *This is just not a dream.*
> *It is our responsibility.*
> James Wolfensohn, President, the World Bank

> *"However secure and well-regulated civilized life may become, bacteria, protozoa, viruses, infected fleas, lice, ticks, mosquitoes, and bedbugs will always lurk in the shadows ready to pounce when neglect, poverty, famine, or war lets down the defenses. And even in normal times they prey on the weak, the very young and the very old, living along with us, in mysterious obscurity waiting their opportunities."*
> Hans Zinsser, 1878-1940

Chapter One

The Universal Declaration of Human Rights and Global Health

Historical Background

War viewed from any perspective is symptomatic of trauma, generally accompanied by horrific injuries and deformation, hatred, violence, mistrust, victimization, destruction, displacement of people, survival, and the ultimate, death. The Second World War or World War II (WW 2) was no exception and was the most widespread war in the history of mankind. It involved a titanic conflict for domination, starting with Germany's invasion of Poland on September 1, 1939, without prior warning, and culminating subsequently in the formation of military alliances led by Nazi Germany, Italy, and Japan known as the Axis. The other war alliance known as the Allies, were led by the United Kingdom, France, the Soviet Union and the United States, and fully intent to stop the objectives of the Axis alliance. Historians of the war reported, interestingly, that each country got engaged in the war on their own

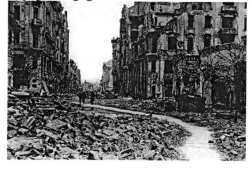

accord, presumably based on their individual outlook/convictions of the conflict and how it would affect their interests, concept of governance, political philosophy, and the overall impact of the war, both short-term and long-term on their own countries.

The fighting involved more than 100 million personnel from the different countries, and indirectly impacted more than a billion people worldwide. Every country used resources to the fullest – human, scientific, economic, and industrial to the war effort. In the process, over seventy million perished, sadly, mostly civilians, making World War II, the deadliest conflict in man's history. Hitler's barbaric onslaught of the Jews during the war was a tragic circumstance of the conflict and caused the deaths of millions of Jews, Gypsies, and mentally handicapped in the concentration camps of Nazi Germany. This aspect of the war was a distinct insult to the world's conscience. The war ended in 1945 with the surrender and defeat of the Axis alliance, and a retrospective assessment of the circumstances that led to the barbaric crimes and oppression were immediately taken to avoid future occurrences of the same nature from ever taking place again.

The world was temporarily paralyzed by shock and indignation. The atrocities, annihilation, and mere decency, including a cry for justice, stimulated the need for a Universal Declaration of Human Rights that would hopefully preclude the likelihood of a recurrence of the indignities of war. Obviously, other factors were involved in the genesis and formatting of the "Declaration," but the atrocities associated with the treatment of the Jews stood out as the clarion call for justice and became the central focal point to the effort of the writing of the Declaration.

Many world leaders, academics, historians, and influential journalists were also of the opinion that the Holocaust perpetuated by the Nazis against European Jewry was paramount in changing the worldview of human rights. Human rights prior to World War II and the behavior of Nazi Germany during the war were never considered from a global perspective. Rights were traditionally considered private and national in scope, in essence, a domestic matter to be handled at a local level and normally limited to a nation and their traditional customs. Rightfully, that ended in 1948 with the Universal Declaration of Human Rights to address the widespread and horrendous wrongs and indignities inflicted on a people during warfare.

The Universal Declaration of Human Rights: Applicability to Poverty and Health

We should remember that the history of civilization has addressed rights from every conceivable perspective, or, at least, by distinct inferences, including the bible and other religious documents. The references for comparative discussion in this text are major written declarations that have had worldwide impact. While not specific to our objective, the United States Declaration of Independence adopted in July, 1776 is an exemplar: "We hold these truths to be self-evident, that all men are created equal, that they are endowed by their Creator with certain unalienable Rights, among these are Life, Liberty, and the pursuit of Happiness." The world has grown to consider this the crux of Abraham Lincoln's political philosophy, and something that influenced America and its people over the years, leading up to the abolition of slavery.

France, about 12 years after the United States, in 1789, developed their country's Declaration of the Rights of Man and of the Citizen that proposed: "the rights of Man are universal; valid at all times and in every place, pertaining to human nature itself." This all took place during the French Revolution and a clear response of the emerging political principles of the Age of Enlightenment at the time. These two important declarations, one from the old world, and the other, the new world, preceded the Universal Declaration of Human Rights, the global template, by over 170 years.

The reference to World War II in this book and the brief history and rationale for the "Declaration" was only meant to provide a transformation and connectedness to the totality of rights, especially the considerate applicability of some of the 30 Articles of the document, and the philosophy of the principle thoughts outlined about 65 years ago in the Declaration to the problems facing global health today. Hopefully, select segments of the document can serve

3

as an absolute set of guidelines or potential "commandments," that we can benefit from and help global health decision makers and advocates to establish another mantra for decency and action by incorporating and highlighting common values that all peoples of the world could mutually aspire to with an objective to promote equity, justice, alleviate poverty and conquer hunger, and, in the process, improve health globally, especially for the vulnerable populations most at risk living in developing countries in a jungle of hopelessness. The ultimate goal, then, is to treat disease control and health, including the opportunities to obtain basic health care as a right for all people in a spirit of brotherhood and social and health security.

Many of the articles in the Universal Declaration address directly and indirectly aspects of life, living, well-being, dignity, equity, social justice, economics, and health. These will be examined contextual to standards of living and the environment, poverty, education, governance, malnutrition/hunger, disease prevalence, and aspects and concepts of the provision of primary health care as a corrective force in preventing disease and promoting health.

The Relevance of the Preamble and Specific Articles of the Declaration

The Universal Declaration of Human Rights was an historic act and a distinct accomplishment by its adoption by the United Nations Assembly in 1948. The theme and direction of the declaration was fully articulated in the first two lines of the preamble: "Whereas recognition of the inherent dignity of the equal and inalienable rights of all members of the human family is the foundation of freedom, justice and peace in the world"....... It was a triumph for the unification of ideals to highlight human dignity and brotherhood throughout a world that was just recovering from the decimation and destruction of war. It provided a broad vista for hope and a new beginning for better tomorrows for a world craving for change.

While just about every article of the declaration has varying degrees of validity in heightening the concept of equality in dignity and rights, four articles are highlighted for relevance to health and well-being:

Article 3 - Everyone has the right to life, liberty and security of person.

Article 5 – No one shall be subjected to torture or to cruel, inhuman or degrading treatment or punishment.

Article 22 – Everyone, as a member of society, has the right to social security and is entitled to realization, through national effort and international co-operation and in accordance with the organization and resources of each State, of the economic, social and cultural rights indispensable for its dignity and the free development of his personality.

Article 25 – (1) Everyone has the right to a standard of living adequate for the health and well-being of himself and of his family, including food, clothing, housing and medical care necessary for social services, and the right to security in the event of unemployment, sickness, disability, widowhood, old age or other lack of livelihood in circumstances beyond its control.

(2) Motherhood and childhood are entitled to special care and assistance. All children, whether born in or out of wedlock, shall enjoy the same social protection.

Eight words of Article 27, "to share in scientific advancement and its benefits" while philosophically utopian and amplifies good intent, faces the barrier that uplifting language is seldom or never the prevailing experience in developing countries. The sad truth is that quite often words are nothing but words. The educated elite and well-informed in developing countries understand that quite well. The reality is that many returning health care professionals from academic or training institutions in developed countries and the future influencers of change return to their home countries with dreams and aspirations to do great things and make a difference. Most often the hurdles and burden of working with limited facilities and outdated equipment put a death sentence to the dreams. This frustrating realization covers every aspect of medical practice from diagnostics, treatment regimens/interventions to disease control and prevention and research. There are or will be some obvious exceptions in some countries and that should be celebrated, but the consensus is that scientific advancement and benefits are not really shared equitably in developing countries, especially in the rural areas that continue to suffer from the lack of development and supporting infrastructure to meet the existing needs or demands of the people.

The different movements and programs for shared cooperation and collaboration in global health provide rays of hope for advances in the many health initiatives that are taking place, but bridging the gap of technological medical advances between the developed and developing countries will take decades to accomplish. The truth is that most of the inequalities that take place in individual countries, and globally, show that the benefits of medical, scientific, and public health advances predominate for some and seldom or never enjoyed by others. This once again illuminates that human rights declarations and covenants will not bring an end to the current and future urgent need for food, vaccines, medical services, good housing, jobs, better education, and improved governance to curtail violations of basic human rights, health or otherwise, for impoverished people.

Articles 3, 5, and 22 fully highlight some of the important basic aspects and concepts of life and living, and the role of society through national efforts to establish economic, social and cultural rights for the development of people. These facets become directly and indirectly ingrained in the goals to achieve hopeful changes that would improve the lives and living conditions of millions of people worldwide, and provide opportunities for the mitigation of poverty, hunger, and disease – forces that remain serious deterrents to global health progress, particularly in low income resource countries that impact billions of people worldwide.

While these articles (3, 5, and 22) serve and contribute to definite attributes that promote fundamentals to improve standards of living and social progress that are integral to health, article 25 exemplifies more specifically the heart of the health-related issues

Don A. Franco

during the formatting of the Universal Declaration in 1948. This article will examine the interlude defined in the Universal Declaration and the forces leading up to the objectives defined 30 years later in 1978 in the World Health Organization's Health for All 2000 program promoting primary health care objectives as a most worthy considerate option for global health. The message is that health concerns have been integral to a global policy agenda for decades, and continue to be a challenging dilemma for decision makers as we look in retrospect to where we have been and where we plan to go in the future.

The global health community and decision makers could definitely benefit from the advice of Yogi-ism, as prescribed by the ultimate satirist, Yogi Berra, who advised: "When you come to the fork in the road, take it." The global health path of the future is circuitous and full of forks in the road. Success will definitely depend on how well the leaders in global public health take those forks in the road and apply them to the long-term strategies to benefit mankind's health globally. As we attempt to take those forks in the road, we would do well to stop and seek advice and direction from those at roadside looking on but treading our same path with doubts, but hope. They are the most affected by the policies that emerge from decision-making and are doubtless hoping that we arrive at our destination with new workable options and goals that could lead to solutions. The vulnerable and those most at risk are waiting at the fork in the road and wondering whether the decisions made would truly reflect their interests and assist their well-being and path to better health.

Article 25 was also clear in intent for the health and well-being of mankind, addressing medical care and social services including food, clothing, housing and the right to security. And, in circumstances that are uncontrollable like unemployment, sickness, disability, and old age, the availability of services to address the needs of the people.

The thought that more than six decades after the adoption of the Universal Declaration of Human Rights promoting the principles of common values that respect freedoms, we are still witnessing the deliberate extermination of peoples in some regions of the world, civil wars with the concurrent rape and assault of women and young girls, the displacement of people resulting from various forms of conflict, the continuing inequalities and rampant poverty, hunger, and disease in poor countries, begging the question, where are the rights of these people? This is not meant as an indictment of the governance of the United Nations, and the world's political leadership in general, other than for all concerned to examine again the whys of limited progress and obvious failure, pronouncedly so in the least developed countries. Why are we so far from realizing the benefits of all the ideals expressed in the declaration? What went wrong? When are we going to regroup to assure the spirit, progress, and success of one of the best written forward looking documents is truly realized? Are more declarations the answer? Is there an answer to this continuing demise? Can global declarations work in a world characterized by marked inequities?

Unfortunately, declarations like the Universal Declaration are sadly unenforceable, and at the dawn of the 21st century too many living in developing countries have neither an understanding nor appreciation of rights, nor do they truly benefit from the rights that were meant to promote social security for the world's least fortunate populations. Optimists can rightly claim with supporting evidence that there has been a remarkable amount of progress in developing countries since the adoption of the declaration in 1948. The world today, however, continues to be full of mostly discouraging news that mock and defy our collective goodwill and ingenuity, and emerging threats will likely remain a distinct challenge to the mostly poor of all developing countries.

Is Health Care Truly A Right?

Rights have been a part of international debates from the advent of civilization from diverse perspectives, and, doubtless, will continue to be an integral part of the ongoing debates nationally and globally for years to come. The right to health care is central to that debate. Even an advanced and enlightened society like the United States, while advancing the basic rights of equity and fairness, still is in the midst of examining considerate options for the universal provision of health care for the country. The subject is complex and contentious, loaded with logical pros and cons from supporters of some form of health coverage for all, and those who are opposed based on the heightened fear that a government-run health care programs would be poorly administered, inefficient and bureaucratic and that people should have the right to choose their health options through the complex maze of existing programs and health insurance. It would be difficult to find someone in the Congress of the United States, regardless of what people think of politicians in general, who would not advocate that people have a right to a standard of living adequate for health and well-being. That analogy is not the issue. It is how the provision of health care services is to be accomplished that is at the heart of the matter. That continues to be the current cause of the ongoing division, both political and philosophical that is taking place throughout the country. The points – counter points reach titanic dimensions at times, emotionally charged, and often appear beyond hope of rational discourse, denying opportunities for either cooperation or collaboration for the mature and academic assessment of health policies and needs of the population.

Interestingly, as debates continue in the global health care arena, it becomes apparent that a constant in every country of the world is that there remain challenging problems in every system. Health care horrors continue to exist in some of the wealthiest countries with the greatest technological advances, and there is an immense continuous effort in most advanced societies to curtail the rising cost of care. This necessitates that many countries are continually studying varying measures of health care reform to counter the existing challenges only to frustratingly recognize that regardless of how efficient a health care system is there will still be widespread dissatisfaction and complaints. This is a paradox. Equally paradoxical is that regardless of the budget for health care, many doctors and hospitals, even in well-resourced settings, will argue that money spent is insufficient and not enough to truly meet the established health care objectives.

Regardless of the aspects and concepts of health care and what side of the debate you are on, the United States is the only advanced and wealthy society without a system of universal health care. This reverts to the rationale for the current model of health care promoted by the United States that is based on experience and the opinion that the private sector is far superior at managing any form of business venture better than government can, and that includes the management of the health of the nation. The opposing view of many in this contentious debate is that Medicare that pays for basic health care for the elderly is government administered and has been and remains a very well managed program overall based on historical assessments with administrative costs of only about 3 percent.

On the night of March 21, 2010, the United States Congress passed a bitterly fought health care reform bill along ideological lines, with the slim margin of 219-212, with no Republicans supporting the bill. The bill's passage brought a likely semblance of universal coverage of health care to Americans for the first time. The vote came at a time that even proponents concede that the legislation as proposed had flaws. President Obama, and the Democratic majority in Congress, nonetheless, was of the opinion that the legislation was a political mandate and a move in the right direction ensuring health care coverage for 95% of Americans.

The close Congressional battle in the passing of the bill characterizes the existing tension and distrust in American society about the provision of health care in general and reverts to rights in the discourse of health policies. Michael Tomasky reporting in the United Kingdom's Guardian the day after the contentious vote was philosophical about some of the prevailing sentiments in the United States and highlighted some of the underlying tensions of people, amplifying some of the expressed concerns of people - whether people should be left alone to pursue their self interest in health care as they have traditionally done or whether or not we should act like a community of citizens with mutual ties and obligations.

Doubtless, this debate will continue in the future since many aspects of the bill will be phased in over a period of years. The legislation, however, does constitute a form of re-making of health care in the United States and a definite reform of the present system from varied perspectives. Since the vote was likely one of the most divisive with flaring passions and very strong opinions on either side, political healing will have to become a part of the process if there is going to be chance for meaningful progression. Many readily concede that many Americans are not getting what they need in health care, but others feel equally convinced that why that might be true, government's interference in health care is not the solution. The future and the impact of health delivery and the health infrastructure emanating from the passage of this bill will become a part of the country's historical health record. Success or failure, therefore, will be dependent on time, and we wait with interest as elements of the bill are implemented within the established timeframe, or repealed in part or in its entirety as some advocate as necessary.

Will the Right to Health Ever Truly Apply to Developing Countries?

The transmission of diseases, and the emergence of epidemics and pandemics, can no longer be viewed as local problems or predominant to developing countries, but must be viewed as distinct threats to all who inhabit our globe. Drought, earthquakes/tsunamis, crop failures, poverty, hunger, and disease continue to affect the lives of members of the global community, directly and indirectly. These happenings, regrettably, tend to occur more frequently in some parts of the world that are ill-equipped to respond, and relatively resource-poor, lacking infrastructure, governance capabilities, and contributing to a form of subliminal instability that persists in so many developing countries. Nonetheless, because we are all affected, the collective response should be both compassionate and humanistic. The global community has shown and continues to demonstrate its willingness to do so, and this speaks well for the recognition that the dignity of human life, well-being, and health, has no boundaries and should be respected. The haves must continue to show great empathy for the have-nots.

The advent of the 21st century clearly illuminates the scientific, technological, and medical/public health advances that have taken place, hitherto, never before anticipated or experienced in our history. This beneficial development should introduce the opportunities for cooperation and collaboration globally to promote value choices for the alleviation of poverty, hunger, control and prevention of diseases, including constructs to enable a world to indulge in peaceful harmony and the maximization of the potential for promoting rights in all their dimensions for each individual.

This progressivism, however, must recognize the continuing tragedy that over 30,000 children die every day because of the indignity of poverty, malnutrition/hunger, and preventable diseases. The majority of these deaths persist in children who are born into families with nothing, and in families unable to provide the basic necessities for life and living – food, clothing, comfort, shelter, and health needs. Those who do survive these pathologies of poverty, their futures fully resemble those of their parents. This cycle of poverty and its effects tend to remain constant in a cohort of over 3 billion people globally, predominantly domiciled in developing countries. Thus, the varied declarations and pronouncements about the attribution of the rights to health and human dignity, while important, uplifting, and forward-looking are not enough. They are merely words that must translate into action if the mission/vision of better tomorrows for the world's destitute is going to be realized.

One would have to be extremely naïve and a blind believer of dreams to entertain any realistic hopes that the theme of the Universal Declaration describing some of the most basic rights of man, including the right to food, clothing, and medical care could ever become a reality in the 21st century. I am reminded of the critical cynic who in a response to the WHO's health for all 2000 initiative, said with succinct sarcasm, that the goal should have been health for all in 2000 years. Regardless of what side of the ongoing debate that you are on, the indicators illustrate the strong division of opinions on where we are in the complex world of global health, and whether or not we could ever generate the resources needed to provide basic health services to meet the needs of billions in developing countries.

The symptoms of social pathology are so ubiquitous – poverty, excessive infant mortality, widespread malnutrition, poor and inadequate delivery of health care, lack of jobs, infrastructural deficits, and poor governance – collectively kill any hope of optimism. Ironically, and with some satire, in developed countries many die from conditions due to excessive intake of food, while more than a billion people in the world go to bed hungry every night. Paradox has a face!

The right to health and medicine, in general, are so divorced from current reality that regrouping of the global health leadership is a mandate for instituting correctives. It is impossible to move the agenda toward health and medical rights without correcting the existing inequalities of social development and economic growth. It should be granted that governments in many developing countries are forming collaborative alliances to act and respond to the needs of the governed, but mostly continue to utterly fail to make any impact on the destitute sick of their populations. Albeit, there are exceptions and some limited cause for optimism. But, the immensity of the challenge to bring programs to reform and remediate inequalities to assure that all humans can lead free and healthy lives is downright defying, and really shows no light that the right to health in developing countries will be attained in any of the timeframes established by proponents of global health reform programs. This dilemma exists in spite of all the progressive programs that are successful and ongoing in so many countries. And, doubtless, for years to come, we will still need interventions throughout the developing world to correct the health care inequalities that could assist mankind to be healthy and free.

Discussion

Why is a new global health perspective needed becomes once again a logical and poignant question. One immediate answer is because despite all our draconian efforts to reform the health care system globally, we continue to be in the milieu of changing challenges that have become more defying and complex devoid of clear directions or satisfying solutions. We are still grappling with failure of many of the articles in the Universal Declaration that specifically addressed issues like freedom, justice, peace, social progress, dignity, liberty, and security written about 65 years ago. Additionally, Health for All by the Year 2000 was the euphoric aspiration that started in Alma Ata (Kazakhstan) during a Conference on Primary Health Care (PHC) in 1978. The objective was to permit people throughout the planet to lead a socially and economically productive life. The prevailing philosophy was that health is a basic human right and that health resources need to be equitably distributed between and within countries. Disappointingly, in spite of the utmost of best intentions, the goals of Health for All 2000 fell short of expectations and remain a definite affront to global health practice.

As early as 1994, a World Health Organization (WHO) review team determined that the health for all by 2000 initiative could not be accomplished. This again triggers a logical concern, why do some of the greatest declarations and objectives to improve the lives of people throughout the world fail? Unless, that question is answered and resolved, future initiatives could also never be realized and would likely continue to fail. The limitations of progressivism that have been ongoing for decades must be debated and resolved by all with a concerted interest in poverty, hunger, disease control and prevention and the promotion of health.

The Millennium Development Goals (MDGs) have now become the new "epistle" to bring new life into equity, social justice, and primary health care initiatives to heighten the attributes of globalization and serve as an impetus to improve the health of the world's least fortunate people. Unfortunately, and, again, in spite of the bold and ambitious plans to uplift the lives of deprived people, current indicators are that many of the defined objectives would not be realized within the 2015 timeframe established for completion.

Overall progress in global health, therefore, continues to be unequal, and many developing countries show no signs of measurable gains. The limited progress of many of the established goals, compounded by unforeseen crises throughout the world could lump MDGs into the same sad fate as the Universal Declaration of Human Rights and the Health for All 2000 initiative. This could be a serious setback for the global health momentum when so many organizations and dedicated people are truly committed to make the world a better place for all. We need no more failed programs and movements. Global health now needs small bites at a time and a new agenda devoid of the all embracing objectives of Health for All 2000 and the Millennium Development Goals, as worthy and well-intentioned the objectives of those two programs were. It is quite conceivable that past endeavors were too much, with too little, in too short of a time. The world is far too complex and unpredictable for grand designs that are longitudinal in scope, even when the formula for success in the development of the goals seemed so applicable and achievable during the initial planning stages.

We must not think that we live in a world overtaken by darkness without hope. Serious challenges exist and would continue to be issues for many years if we hope to have a progressive agenda for change. Something as elemental as the global health community's examination of determinants of health, especially in resource poor countries remains fraught with frustration for strategic planning of programs. The basic data needed for making intelligent decisions are unreliable, deficient, and nothing more than mere estimates. While primary health care is promoted as the logical option, there is no workable or reliable system in place to determine whether care in all of the developing countries is continuous or effective. The mere lack of registration systems in most poor countries for the recording of births and deaths remains a serious public health deterrent. This continues in the 21st century when that type of information is a fundamental factor in decision making for the public health infrastructure nationally and globally. As correctives go, this must become a priority.

Global estimates are that two thirds of all deaths are not registered. In essence mortality statistics that are so necessary for health planning objectives are mostly unobtainable. In fact, WHO is only able to obtain cause of death information from 31 of the almost 200 Member States of the United Nations. These deficiencies are so much a part of the challenging dilemma of the pathologies of poverty and the lack of governance that continue to exist in the poor countries of the world. Even vital statistics, so fundamentally necessary for coordinating, collaborating, and determining the future objectives for health care contribute to the litany of elementary deficiencies that stymie progress. In an era where information technology, the computer, and the Internet has become a part of daily use, developing countries must make every effort and apply this form of technological advancement to benefit governance that could ultimately assist strategic planning efforts to improve services and build on infrastructure. Some of these improvements could be worked out with donor organizations, both governmental and private/non-profit and are often not cost-prohibitive.

Caution is in order. Many well-meant suggestions that appear relatively simple to those willing to assist poor countries get to another tier could be fraught with greater challenges that are not readily understood by those extern to the daily realities and happenings of resource-poor countries. While data collection seems readily doable and simple, like in the case of a corrective approach for informatics involving vital statistics, the forces at work in developing countries could make the change initiative a real challenge and more complex than initially realized. Common sense should prevail. An information system could be easily devised by delegating decisions to the people who will implement them, and then gather only information that is necessary for decision making. Unfortunately, quite often, the circumstances in many bureaucracies of developing countries cannot adjust to what appear to be a logical, simple and beneficial change. The infrastructure, most of the time, simply cannot support change, regardless of the perceived benefits; so goals, especially those developmental in scope and necessitating change have to be contextual and would vary from country to country and dependent on resources.

Rights have been debated from every conceivable perspective from the advent of civilization and will likely continue to be discussed globally as a sphere of social intercourse and health promotion objectives for years in the future. Regardless of the goals of declarations and interpretations of them, one theme must prevail to demonstrate that all people should have certain basic rights to conform to the "inherent dignity and of the equal and inalienable rights of all members of the human family" and that should serve as "the foundation of freedom, justice, and peace in the world....to promote social progress and better standards of life in larger freedom......that every individual and organ of society shall strive by teaching and education to promote respect for these rights and freedoms and by progressive measures, national and international, to secure their universal and effective recognition and observance..." Inherent dignity and inalienable rights of the human family can ill afford the continuing indignity and hopelessness of poverty, hunger, and disease that devastate more than half of the world's population of over three billion people in the 21st century.

While some of the expressed concerns seem tentative and indicting, there are lights of encouragement and hope with cause for celebration on the progress in many spheres of global health. The eradication of smallpox is an icon in the history of global health accomplishments and could become a model for other efforts to eliminate or eradicate other vaccine preventable diseases. The success in global childhood vaccinations in general, including polio, provides a great deal of encouragement for the future. There is epidemiological evidence that dracunculiasis (guinea worm disease) is close to eradication. This exemplifies the role of private foundations like the Carter Center that led the charge with the

17

unification of collaborating forces to make this disease no longer the debilitating threat it has been for centuries in many African countries.

The African Program for Onchocerciasis (River Blindness) Control highlights the benefits of collaboration with the pharmaceutical industry (in this case Merck) to assist communities to conduct their own treatment programs with the drug mectizan (ivermectin) for more than 46 million people. The continuing progress in the prevention efforts and treatment of HIV/AIDS through effective antiretroviral therapy has amplified the political will to confront the disease on a worldwide basis with donor assistance. Serious challenges continue to serve as barriers; the control of tuberculosis and malaria remains defying, especially in resource-poor countries, but the public health success of the aforementioned infectious diseases provides lights of encouragement.

Infectious diseases are exemplified, for obvious reasons – they have historically demanded and received attention globally because of high morbidity and mortality, compared to the control of chronic diseases that lack the dramatization, including the political sensitivity and visibility, and potential threats to public health, nationally and globally. The severe acute respiratory syndrome (SARS), and other emerging zoonoses like H5N1 avian influenza, the Nipah virus, H1N1 ("swine flu") amplify the concerns of the emerging virulence of pathogens linked to globalization. We, therefore, face the additional global public health threat to respond to new emerging diseases due to the large scale movement of people. Disease is never static, so the challenges to public health throughout the world will continue to test our ingenuity and will.

A recent publication, Real Collaboration – What It Takes for Global Health to Succeed (Rosenberg, Hayes, McIntyre, and Neill – University of California Press) provides illumination and hope to the global health challenges, and had a provocative comment on the cover by an icon in international affairs and global health, former

President Jimmy Carter – "This book addresses one of the major problems facing global health: leadership without cooperation."

Our past failures, whether through written declarations or policy pronouncements, poor management, lack of resources, or simply no directional impetus and indifference, should not deter us from taking that fork in the road once more to benefit mankind. Dr. William (Bill) H. Foege, a public health internationalist, scholar, thinker, motivator, teacher, and leader in health innovations around the globe described optimism in the preface in Real Collaboration that could move us forward with a new sense of renewed zeal and determination:

"We have never been in a better position to extend a hand to people around the globe. With the resources of United Nations agencies, the foundations endowed by Rockefeller, Gates, Buffet, and Turner; Rotary International; pharmaceutical companies; bilateral; multilaterals; and thousands of non-governmental organizations, we have an abundance to tap that is beyond anything we could have imagined fifty years ago. And the most important lesson of those fifty years is that collaboration is the best way to make those resources count. Real collaboration. The give-and-take of human beings who are so dedicated to a mission they will set aside the politics of organizations, share the difficulties, and invent solutions together.......As we take these steps to build the discipline of collaboration into our work, we also need to show respect for our partners from the developing world, from government, from NGOs, or from the private sector. They are the ones who could teach us to move forward. Medical knowledge is not enough. Western leadership is not enough. Money is not enough. We must depend on each other. Only with respect for what all of us can contribute will we understand the best way to approach global health threats. Only then can we use the abundant resources available in a way that opens up the possibility of global health equity in the twenty-first century." --- AMEN!!

Bill Foege has already allowed so many to stand on his shoulders and look at the world and see what can be done to improve the lot of the many destitute who are hollering to be cared for and desperately looking for better tomorrows. His inspirational guidance should provide impetus and a true sense of direction to all who share his dreams to make life and living a universal experience of human dignity for all peoples and all nations.

Conclusion

The aforementioned discourse examined aspects of the Universal Declaration of Human Rights from an historical perspective, its applicability to poverty, well-being, and health, the relevance and pertinence of specific articles of the declaration, the concept of health care being a right, and an assessment whether the right to health can ever truly apply or be achieved in developing countries. Reflections of the 1978 health for all by the year 2000 initiative, and the current Millennium Development Goals (MDGs) program were heightened contextual to the historical overview of where we have been, and where we plan to go, and how we plan to get there. These subjects will be presented in more detail in specific chapters.

The authors of the declaration attempted to format and affirm broad aspects of social, cultural, and economic rights by setting high goals. That we have failed to meet them is no reason to abandon hope or become discouraged. We must continue to dream that one day we could all enjoy a common standard of equal and inalienable rights, including the right to health, regardless of the compelling hurdles that will entail.

We must all pursue, as members of the global community, a common objective to help governments throughout the world to improve their public health infrastructure to meet the needs of their populations, especially for the most vulnerable and destitute of society. This necessitates a successful end to the widespread inequalities to health care services by optimizing and maximizing the attributes of public health science for the world's poorest communities. The techniques of the past have failed, and we are in

20

urgent need of a new agenda for instituting change and reform if we are true believers that global health is indeed central to social justice. We must join the mobilization for continuing change. The global health challenges are so widespread and complex that no single player has the capability to do it alone. We need one another more than ever in this elusive climate for meaningful change if we have any chance of having a sustained impact on billions of people globally.

The ubiquitous poverty of most developing countries, including the paucity of an economic and health infrastructure precludes the building of a framework that will provide health sustainability. No two countries are truly alike, even though some have distinct commonalities and challenges that parallel, demanding that strategic plans to be workable must consider the unique and distinct characteristics of each country. Many countries have made genuine attempts to embrace science-based care strategies to their programs, but most remain in diverse forms of transition because of their inability to develop a single system to adapt to population needs. The result is a myriad of disorganized systems with different approaches to care varying from traditional to public or private type clinics or hospitals.

This lack of coordination and organization of the existing medical resources contributes to a lack of uniformity and poor performance. This serves as a deterrent to improving the health status of communities, reducing inequalities, increasing efficiencies, and enhancing fairness. One generic consideration that could have broad applicability to many developing countries is the establishment of health centers and hospitals that are responsive to the health needs of the locals, and, would serve the collective disease control and primary health care goals of individual countries. This could be the starting point for real collaboration and the dream of ultimate success to make health care for all a reality in the future, even in a "climate" of extreme barriers and hurdles necessitating will, commitment, strategic planning, and good governance.

Every day that we fail to act compounds the problem. The response does not have to be grandiose or all-inclusive like some of the approaches of the past six decades that failed to meet the sought after outcomes or materialize to the fullest. They could be modest, and, most often should be, because of limited resources, provided they meet the needs of the people. The time to do so is now!!! Plan strategically, communicate openly, indulge the masses that would be impacted by the decision making, maximize transparency, coordinate efficiently, and collaborate with passion to achieve the established objectives. Optimize the virtues of real collaboration in the process, and empower dedicated people who are committed to work for change. Success will be ours. Failure is not an option.

"Events of massive, public suffering defy quantitative analysis. How can one really understand statistics citing the death of six million Jews or graphs of third-world starvation? Do numbers really reveal the agony, the interruption, the questions that these victims to the meaning and nature of our individual lives and life as a whole?
Rebecca Chopp, The Praxis of Suffering

"There is, of course, plenty of (poverty) in the world in which we live. But more awful is the fact that so many people – including children from disadvantaged backgrounds – are forced to lead miserable and precarious lives and to die prematurely. That predicament relates in general to low incomes, but not just to that. It also reflects inadequate public provisions and nutritional support, deficiency of social security arrangements, and the absence of social responsibility and of caring governance."
Amartya Sen, Mortality as an Indicator of Economic Success and Failure

Chapter 2

"Health for All" By the Year 2000: A Retrospective Analysis

Historical Background

In a world of about six and a half billion people, and approximately 200 countries, health care debates have been constant over the years. The discussions became especially acute and relevant during the period of the 1960s and 1970s, particularly in developing countries, when many nations in Africa and the Caribbean region became newly independent states. Many of these countries wanted to demonstrate their new status and heighten their responsibility and accountability post-colonialism to the new challenges of governing by modifying and attempting fundamental changes to their health care delivery system. One considerate option in the new direction and approach was to promote equity, and move from the traditional and highly practiced curative aspects of health care to disease control and prevention programs that embrace the principles of primary health care which were coming to age at the time in many developed countries with encouraging results.

A few countries were tentative and established commissions and task force type assessments to evaluate future objectives and initiatives for the direction of their health programs. In fact, the period could be considered one of opportunistic transition for reform; not only in health policies, but other spheres of social advancement including the intent for improved governance and the concurrent building of infrastructure, a need of all developing countries. It was also the ideal period and environment to show changed leadership, a sense of autonomy, and a feel for true independence in decision making by the new governments. Like most transitions, the path was not well defined or orderly, other than change was, indeed, a new right, and demonstrating the ability to pursue and consider reform was an action that would be viewed favorably by the populations served. Additionally, one likely advantage in the transformational thinking was a purging of some of the dictates and traditions of the colonial past, whether or not they had distinct attributes. It was the right time for the consideration of new options and to demonstrate independence, and health care reform was a logical opportunity to do so in a rapidly changing world.

Change was the new norm that should be embraced. Since health care was always a part of the debate in most, if not all developing countries, prudence would dictate that any form of change was a safe venture to pursue politically, since it was likely to be viewed positively by both consumers of health care and governments responsible for the provision of care, including the professional leadership anxious to show their ability to govern and manage. This transformation was obviously not limited to the newly independent countries, but seemed a symptom of responding to the changing needs of populations in mostly resource-poor countries and a counter alternative to the rising cost of health care services in many of these countries.

At or around this time, international organizations like the World Health Organization (WHO), had started to consider new directions for delivery of health care in developing countries to heighten equity

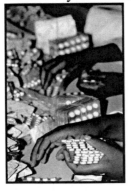 and the promotion of disease prevention as the most applicable and cost-effective consideration. Interestingly, at the advent of the 21st century, we are still promoting equity, and it is most likely that will continue to be a continuing objective for years to come, possibly forever in some countries. That aside, the vision for health care services in the future seemed fully geared toward prevention in lieu of the traditional curative practices. That emerging philosophy was a good start because

so much more could be accomplished by the instituting of good public health practice and prevention programs, including the greater cost-benefits derived in the process, provided sustainability was also a strategic objective. That has been affirmed by longitudinal studies in many developed countries as being more cost-effective, providing impetus for decision makers in developing countries for their new objectives.

A Correlation of China's Health for the Masses and "Health for all 2000"

During the 1960s, China had to start a serious program to meet the health care demands of its burgeoning population. That was a problematic undertaking for the country with both doctors and money in short supply. There was also the additional urgent need to combat widespread infectious diseases that plagued the country, especially among the peasantry, and those living in the rural areas of the country. With a ready supply of people in the rural regions of the country, and the concurrent launching of the Cultural Revolution around that period, China's governing leadership under the Chairmanship of Mao Zedong, decided to make health reform a part of the "Great Leap Forward" that the country needed. This decision for health reform necessitated the training of a cadre of predominantly young people, mostly peasants, to assist this novel initiative. Those selected were given rudimentary education in the basics of health care, highlighting aspects/concepts of sanitation and hygiene, and disease control and prevention to reflect the needs of the rural population. This newly emerged addition to the country's health movement became known as the "barefoot doctors." This name seemed to truly characterize this new force in health promotion because they combined work in the field as peasant farmers with their new responsibilities of providing basic health services to the people.

The role of the "barefoot doctors" supplemented China's existing health infrastructure and contributed to definite improvements in health delivery like immunizations and maternal care, especially in the rural regions that traditionally had limited services. The concept of introducing an intermediary medical support resource like envisioned for the "barefoot doctors" was to serve the basic health care needs of the population in the countryside, mostly poor peasants, but also to sustain signs of economic development in agriculture that had started to be evident by establishing a system of care for the farmers who produce food. Additionally, a clear advantage of this new intervention to reform health services in the country was that the "barefoot doctors" were always available to provide care to the needy, since they lived and worked alongside the people, understood the prevailing problems, and were generally trusted by those they served. The fact that the services were provided at a reduced cost heightened and affirmed the objectives of the government at the time, providing semblances of hope for the improvement and expansion of health services for more people in the future.

Regardless whether China's new health care intervention was a success or not, the World Health Organization (WHO) in its quest to improve and better manage the chronic problems of health care delivery in most developing countries, considered the "barefoot doctor" concept a system that was most worthy of implementing, and likely could apply philosophically to some of the "health for all by 2000" objectives. The thought was that the results experienced in China could apply to nearly all developing countries, especially those with a limited supply of professional and technical support, especially the paucity of doctors. The prevailing enthusiasm was that a "barefoot doctor" system would have distinct applicability for just about all the countries in sub-Saharan Africa, and other resource-poor countries in Asia and Latin America. The problems in sub-Saharan Africa, for example, were so acute that any new intervention would be beneficial with good implementation and governance.

Surprisingly, and with a lot of concurrent interest throughout the globe as to the whys of the decision, China's health planners decided in 1985 that the cooperative medical system that operated mostly at the village level using predominantly the services of the "barefoot doctors" had collapsed and the services they provided would not continue. This included the cancellation of the title "barefoot doctor" to illustrate the new direction of the Ministry of Health. This demise of the health service system for the poor of the countryside was slowly replaced by a free-market pay for health care program that forced peasants to pay for all forms of medical services.

Interestingly, the debate of the functionality of the "barefoot doctors" impact on China's health care continues to this day, about 50 years after it was introduced as the logical response to effectively serve the needs of the farming communities in the rural areas of the country. Many public health authorities throughout the world with an interest in global health innovations and outcomes, while admitting that China's program was by no means without flaws, nonetheless, had effusive praise for the many aspects of the program that at least provided many basic health care services to vast numbers of people, hitherto, who had only very minimal or no health care. Equally encouraging, also, was the convincing evidence that "barefoot doctors" played a very important early role in the reduction of infectious diseases that plagued the country for years. This was done through simple education of the masses about the application of sanitation and hygienic principles, exemplified by the impressive decreased incidence of schistosomiasis, a snail-borne disease that was endemic along river basins of the country. Obviously, the success was not limited to schistosomiasis, but to many other infectious diseases that threatened the people, especially the poor of the rural areas, always the most vulnerable to disease, infectious or otherwise.

The fact that twenty percent of the world's population live in China, constituting about one third of the global poor, gives global health decision makers a legitimate claim and an ideal profile for comparative study for developing and instituting programs and solutions that could contribute to a "health for all" model, particularly geared to serve the needs of developing countries, since the Chinese government has been challenged by serious public health programs over the years.

A lesson learnt could be that in developing countries characterized by poor resources and a paucity of health professionals, an evaluation of how a system or program like China's "barefoot doctors" could serve the health care needs deserves serious consideration. In fact, one could sensibly surmise that is exactly the reason why WHO global health planners thought the program applicable for basic health care provision in many developing countries, and could likely have attributes in a health for all 2000 goal that was being established.

Irony, without doubt, mocks global health in varying degrees. Just about the time, or shortly after WHO was defining objectives for the health for all 2000 initiative, China's leaders decided to abandon the "barefoot doctors" program and move toward a payment-based system of health care. In essence, a marked contrast in health care policy took place in China in a period of about two decades, 1965-1985. One can rightly ask, why a country that espouses community unity and development as a movement and model, and having instituted a program to meet the needs of the masses that appeared to be accepted, would then abandon a service model for primary health care and embrace a pay for service system? It seemed inconsistent to the policies that were traditionally embraced by China; doubtless, China's planners must have had legitimate reasons for their new direction in care.

Equally unpredictable, and heightening the chaos of irony, no one had the slightest suspicion that during this period of instituting change in health care direction globally that individuals had started to be infected by the human immunodeficiency virus (HIV), culminating in a newly defined killer disease, the acquired immunodeficiency syndrome (AIDS). This illuminated the nuances of medicine and public health, affirming the sad realization that the emergence of new diseases like HIV/AIDS transcends man's knowledge and reason.

Don A. Franco

Alma-Ata and the Health Care Declaration

The "health for all" declaration took place in Alma-Ata, Russia (now Kazakhstan) in 1978, and boldly confirmed that access to basic health services was a fundamental right. Parts of the declaration clearly affirmed the directional emphasis and major themes of the conference, and the priorities that emanated from the assembly: "Health, which is a state of complete physical, mental, and social wellbeing, and not merely the absence of disease or infirmity, is a fundamental human right and that the attainment of the highest possible level of health is a most important world-wide social goal whose realization requires the action of many other social and economic sectors in addition to the health sector..........An acceptable level of health for all people of the world by the year 2000 can be attained through a fuller and better use of the world's resources, a considerable part of which is now spent on armaments and military conflicts.................Primary health care is essential health care based on practical, scientifically sound and socially acceptable methods and technology made universally accessible to individuals and families in the community through their full participation and at a cost the community and country can afford to maintain at every stage of their development in the spirit of self-reliance and self-determination ....It is the first level of contact of individuals, the family and community with the national health system bringing health care as close as possible to where people live and work, and constitutes the first element of a continuing health care process."

On a personal observation, when I first read an article on the "health for all by 2000" goals over 30 years ago, I was markedly ambivalent, euphoric beyond description that any assembly would be forward-looking and progressive enough to consider a health agenda for all people in a defiant world of uncertainty, and equally wondering whether or not the declaration was just hyper-inflated wishful thinking for a needed template for global health, the goals of which have no hope of being accomplished. While I thought the

29

agenda was most noble, I also wondered whether or not some members of the decision-making assembly had visited some of the regions of destitution that I had, and whether or not they would have programmed the same goals. I saw a world bleeding and crying for help and health care intervention, but nothing that could be accomplished in a couple of decades or so. The problems were too complex and ubiquitous, and really defied the most worthy intent of declarations. Nonetheless, I had to give the planners of the conference the benefit of the doubt, but concede that it did not alter my ambivalence in any way, even though I am a blind optimist by nature.

I was also philosophical, and that amplified my ambivalence. For example, I thought in very simple terms by begging the question, why did those responsible for formatting an agenda for global health did not consider at the time something as basic and fundamental like clean water for the world, our most precious resource, and a prerequisite to sanitation, hygiene, and health. In support of my thinking and proposal, I considered the many millions of people who have no access to a sustainable supply of safe drinking water. The Millennium Development Goals (MDGs) still have as an objective to cut in half by 2015 the number of people who do not have access to a potable water supply. With the global water supply still a crisis at the advent of the 21st century, should we not have taken small bites at a time, like specific objectives, in lieu of an all-embracing agenda for health promotion. This does not negate in any way the "nobility" of the "health for all 2000" goal, other than to express concern whether optimism suffers from temporary blindness at times in the quest to do good, or whether our planning for the future buries the pain of reality that many of the barriers to global health are insurmountable by the timeframes that were established.

It is very easy to become a part of the culture of complaints, and no objective person or group of people, organized or otherwise, should criticize the collective efforts of a global assembly of nations intent on problem solving, and in recognition that the electrifying immediacy to correct global health inadequacies is acute. The conference at the time was symptomatic of the euphoria that accompanied the eradication of smallpox. The global health community felt empowered and determined to move forward with other new vistas and agendas. They defied barriers and felt that health for all the people of the world was a valid and worthy objective that should be prioritized and pursued with an "all aboard" attitude. There was every reason to be hopeful and positive during this period. The sentiment was that global health deficits could be something of the past, if we all worked in unison by aspiring together to change the structure of health services to embrace the needs of the poor and vulnerable of the world.

Components of a "Health for All" Program

Whether or not health for all, or a similar all-embracing concept of health reform is ideal but impractical, does not preclude the need for a discussion to define and describe the characteristics or constructs of such a program. It has already been recognized by global health authorities that the uncertainty associated with the spread of infectious agents including the continuing threat of emerging microbes into new geographic areas keeps the world's population at risk to both the consequences of infectious diseases and infections that could trigger a chronic disease with the likelihood that some could be linked to cancer. The epidemiological evidence over the years that some chronic diseases have definitely been associated with an infectious etiology e.g. cervical cancer with several papilloma viruses, predominant in developing countries create serious challenges to global health sustainability. The same applies to peptic ulcer disease, and possible stomach cancer linked to Helicobacter pylori, a ubiquitous organism in resource-poor countries. The challenge, therefore, is that efforts to construct any type of "health for all" reform initiative would continue to be burdened by the same barriers faced by past programs. This also includes the current Millennium Development Goals (MDGs) formatted to replace some of the language in the Universal

Declaration of Human Rights and the failures of "health for all by 2000" by the year 2015. In fact, public health pragmatists, who have advocated a global health agenda geared to improving the plight of the poor must wonder why did the well meant and formulated objectives fail, or to be fairer, did not accomplish their targeted goals? Poverty, hunger, and disease continue to defy global health strategists. The so-called "10/90 gap" defined as only 10 percent of global health research is devoted to conditions responsible for 90 percent of the global burden of disease must be a source of concern. The compelling evidence remains that the major diseases of developing countries, distressingly poor and resource deficient, do not receive the proportionate research/medical attention, contributing to an embarrassing imbalance, should be a cause for corrective action. Additionally, and a continuing never ending affront to the ingenuity of global health strategists is that the disease burden in all low income countries is associated with poverty. Three diseases of

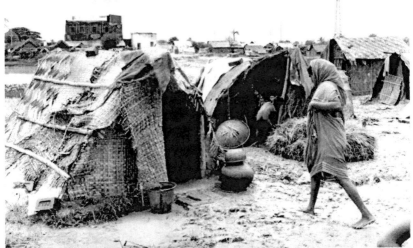

poverty, tuberculosis, malaria, and HIV/AIDS illustrate the dilemma – these diseases account for about 18 percent of the disease burden in the poorest countries. Estimates from another WHO report indicate that 45 percent of the global disease burden is linked to poverty. Especially challenging for all resource-deficient countries is that non-communicable diseases that have traditionally been a serious public health challenge to developed countries like cancer, cardiovascular diseases and neurological diseases now have become a serious medical burden for developing countries. In countries with health care systems still in varying stages of development, this additional yoke is a serious affront to health services.

Where do we go, and how do we proceed in this environment clouded by uncertainty? One glaring challenge is to take once more another look at an all-inclusive global approach that would benefit developing countries and maximize/optimize effectiveness and efficiency to benefit those in need. The reality is that we cannot just give up. A lot of progress has been made in so many spheres of global health. In the midst of darkness, and draconian hurdles there is still hope. The challenges, nonetheless, will remain demanding. The new goals could consider:

1. Eliminate the hyper-inflationary language so traditional of past declarations that promotes idealism and is inspirational but impractical and often defies reality. Program success will depend on the establishment of collaborative alliances with locals to develop health intervention strategies at all activity levels from the small district health clinics serving rural populations to major hospital centers to health ministries and departments involved in policy formulation. This will heighten the role of locals and legitimize long-term efforts by the buy-in involvement and commitment. In the 21st century, foreign technocrats still play a significant part in health development in resource-poor countries, but that must be limited to a team approach and as a part of planned collaboration and not the dictates as was customary in the past.

2. The "for all" approach must be based on existing and future needs of individual countries instead of the all inclusive goals practiced in previous health initiatives. In essence, a regionalization perspective based on assessments.

Concession can be made that commonalities prevail in many of the countries of sub-Saharan Africa, Asia, Latin America, and the Caribbean, but success will only be truly realized through working with individual countries to meet the most challenging health problems through specific corrective interventions. The ideal would be small governable and manageable programs at a local level with responsibility and accountability for outcomes clearly objectified. This should entail onsite and timely evaluations of the goals to be accomplished, and correctives as necessary during the process when goals are not achieved.

3. Eliminate all barriers to health care by making health care free or just token affordable reimbursements for services. No one should ever be turned away because he/she cannot pay the cost of health services. One barrier that must be eliminated especially in the rural areas of all developing countries is inadequate transportation. This can be done through the building of infrastructure and collaboration with government, the private sector, and non-governmental organizations (NGOs) based on assessment of needs and long-term strategic planning. A logical goal and consideration is to build clinics in rural areas to provide health services to those who live in isolated areas heightening access to care.

4. Promote comprehensive care using the principles of primary health care to the fullest by addressing proper nutrition to abate malnutrition and deficiency diseases, the use of educational resources for risk reduction to improve population health by behavior changes, the promotion of immunization/vaccination as a public health imperative, and when applicable joint strategies and collaboration by government, the private sector and NGOs to enhance a healthy lifestyle with emphasis on maternal and child health promotion.

5.   Collaboration with the locals is essential for the success of programs in developing countries and provides empowerment to local organizations, including the professional and support staff, while promoting the advantages of active involvement and "buy-in" needed to progress. This is especially applicable for donor organizations and NGOs intent on establishing health promotion and disease prevention and control initiatives. The active participation of the local leadership adds credence and legitimizes the efforts, and is a perfect example of the benefits of coalition, communication, collaboration, and program continuity to accomplish objectives.

6.   A successful primary health care delivery system mandates coordination of objectives and established goals through health informatics and does not necessarily have to be an expensive undertaking or technologically advanced as used in developed countries. Delegate the decision making as close as possible to the people who would be implementing the programs, and only use information that is necessary for the decisions and progress of the programs. This involves many of the daily activities related to data collection, surveillance, and other logistics related to patient care. In developing countries making processes simple pay huge dividends. It also affirms anecdotal evidence that indicates a properly organized communal response to promote health care programs brings people together and maximizes the results through the working towards a cause to benefit the community. It builds unity and goodwill for a common cause, and enhances social responsibility and accountability.

7.   Ensure quality of care. The continuing problem of many developing countries failing to deliver basic health care services including the maintenance of an adequate supply of medicines continues to be challenging. In many countries the distribution system and storage is outdated and

poorly managed resulting in unnecessary losses. Health care services have not been given the priority necessary to maintain a functioning public health system to provide primary health care services. Staffing and inadequate professional support of programs, paucity of equipment, limited elementary diagnostic capabilities, and poor follow-up of patients contribute to the service deficits.

8. Allocate resources within a country's health care system based on the burden of disease, while still adhering to the fundamentals of primary health care as the thematic objective. Countries still burdened by infectious diseases like HIV/AIDS would obviously use anti-retroviral intervention for curative effect, but must also pursue vigorous control and prevention strategies to counter the spread of the virus. The same principles apply to other communicable and non-communicable diseases – prevention through primary health care.

9. Prioritize prevention in the training of health professionals both in developed and developing countries. In developing countries, the proper use of health centers to institute programs that are comprehensive in scope should be strengthened and consideration should be given to the benefits of using non-professional community aids like housewives to support disease prevention and control programs in the villages and rural areas. Those selected could be given a basic education in the fundamentals of public health similar to what was used in China for the "barefoot doctors." Properly motivated and indoctrinated, these people could be a formidable resource for improving health – administering worm medicine to youngsters, follow up for drug compliance of patients with AIDS and tuberculosis, educate on the benefits of elementary sanitation practices, and as a collaboration resource to the health center.

10. Select programs based on cost-benefits. This is particularly necessary in developing countries with limited resources and poor infrastructure. Surveys continue to show the benefits of clean water; yet, in the 21st century many developing countries have a limited access to a safe drinking water supply, both in rural and urban areas. This impacts any hope to institute proper sanitation. The combination of dirty water and poor sanitation account for the death of at least 5,000 children daily, making it the second largest cause of child mortality. A closing thought as we look at the broad challenging dimensions of health, is clean water a basic human right? Are people unreasonable to expect a supply of clean water from governments?

Recommendations of new goals to address global health deficits with corrective interventions have distinct limits and have to be generic in scope because of future uncertainty and unknown circumstances that could influence any form of recommendations. That by no means implies that global health objectives should not have an agenda and timeframe. But, the experience of past declarations and programs like the Universal Declaration of Human Rights and the health for all by the year 2000, provide reason for caution and a new approach. Incidentally, the results of the Millennium Development Goals (MDGs) to be realized by 2015 amplify the need for an end to inflationary pronouncements and declarations.

Many of the priorities of the future of global health goals highlighted the relevance to developing countries for obvious reasons. The developed countries have had and will continue to have challenges, but generally have a built-in public health infrastructure to respond to the needs of their populations. At least, a working system for responding is in place. A point of interest, nonetheless, is that it is likely that the application and promotion of primary health care, with special emphasis on developing countries, could add to the global health progression and success and could have the added benefit of reforming programs at minimal costs to the health care sector in most countries. Additionally, the philosophy that government and the people, in a wave of true collaboration and togetherness could be innovative and strategically develop initiatives that would best serve the needs of the communities provides hope. In the process, this approach could result in greater equity of health resources and overall improvements in services.

Discussion

Health for all by the year 2000 goals must continue to be a part of the retrospective debate, not as a source of blind criticism for the failures to accomplish many of the objectives, but something to help future policy planners for global health look back on and reflect, learn, and hopefully use as a guidepost for the development of other strategies for health programs that will be developed. Granted, the theme, health for all, was never meant to be taken literally. It was nothing more than a philosophical and progressive periscope for WHO member countries to modify their approaches for the prevention and control of diseases, and build on a system of primary health care programs to make health care accessible to all. It was at the time an all inclusive goal with an "audacity of hope." History, then, can become a guiding light to help circumvent mistakes we have made in the past, and not indulge in blind criticism, but serve as an invaluable resource to avoid the pitfalls experienced by others in health care programming globally for future generations. The historical perspective has a definite place in future planning and should never be marginalized or overlooked, because health, in general, has emerged as an important element of the global agenda and history will help to teach us how to capture information from the global health scene and use it as knowledge to benefit health programs globally.

The entire complex of establishing any type of health system that is holistic and catholic for developing countries, or all countries for that matter, is that tendency toward generalization and the continuing mistake of categorizing countries based on likes, for example, the subject of poverty, or in the case of disease prevalence HIV/AIDS. We so often forget that no two countries are truly alike – each country has its own unique characteristics dominated by history, culture, traditions, religion, economics and governance. This necessitates that in the formatting of a centralized and workable health care model, programs must prioritize the needs and expectations of the people of each country. Granted that geography, needs, and the similarity of objectives could overlap into contiguous countries and be cost-beneficial and effective should not be blatantly overlooked, particularly when there are clear benefits to joint efforts in the development of programs.

The potential for successful joint strategic plans for health could apply to some regions of sub-Saharan Africa, Central America, and the Caribbean basin. The likelihood of success will be greater, however, if goals are manageable, limited by geography, and properly supervised. The logic – keep it simple. This is glaringly the case in developing countries, still building on basic governance and infrastructure, and lacking in technical and professional support, and the other necessary facilities including equipment and information technology resources to efficiently handle complex or challenging initiatives.

In retrospect, everyone associated with global health initiatives had great expectations and hope for the success of health for all 2000, despite the lofty and seemingly impossible goals. Can anyone not truly support a transformation that will improve ways to prevent disease, contribute to a better standard of living, and enhance health, especially among the vulnerable poor of the world? Primary health care was proposed as the logical answer to provide an inexpensive but broad medical service to communities as the first level of intervention in a continuum. The objectives envisioned in this type of care will include health education, safe food and clean water as part of environmental sanitation and hygiene, the provision of needed vaccinations, maternal and child care, treatment of common diseases and injuries, disease surveillance and prevention, the promotion of nutritional programs through education, and providing essential drugs. The aforementioned were cheap and effective ways to provide the most in health care to the many in need.

In essence, the concept of primary health care for all countries was deemed futuristic with special applicability to developing countries. It could create a valuable boost to the entire global health infrastructure while contributing to reforming programs at minimal cost and the maximization of benefits to the populations served. It was a part of the goal to add impetus for government and the governed, the people, to work together in a tide of togetherness to make health care more accessible and equitable and become the core delivery system for resource-poor countries.

We are still examining the impact of primary health care advocacy in developing countries and the apparent failure of many to effectively and efficiently institute the new innovations to meet the emerging needs of their populations. Many leaders simply lack the needed dedication, education, commitment and vision for programs to succeed. There continues to be an ongoing battle for adequate funding, a serious frustration, and priorities are often never clearly defined, contributing to poor outcomes and failure to accomplish goals, assuming any are objectified. Poor management and a lack of structure is a constant challenge and contribute to confusion and no sense of direction in many countries preventing the introduction of needed innovations to serve the compelling needs of people.

Unfortunately, regardless of the health options that will be embraced to address the needs of people, particularly in the developing countries, poverty, the condition of the majority of the global population, was and will continue to remain the major deterrent to health. This will contribute to the continuing crisis to health reform. Poverty, therefore, is the central cause of being ill, and about not being able to get medical attention. It is not being a part of the future. It is a source of powerlessness, lack of freedom, and that sinking feeling of hopelessness. It is a condition that people are dying to escape because it contributes to hunger and disease, the theme of this book.

Conclusion

During the period, starting in the 1960s – 1980s, many developing countries, particularly post-independence, had begun to assess their health care programs. This was also guided by WHO's growing momentum to amplify the benefits of primary health care as the logical option for the delivery of health services in all countries. China's health reform was a point of reference for the period, and a source of fascination and intrigue for many leaders in developing countries. The use of "barefoot doctors" as medical/public health auxiliaries was a novel approach, especially in the promotion of health, and the prevention and control of diseases in the rural areas of the country. This was a definite attractant for many developing countries.

Decision makers in the field of public health medicine in some developing countries saw the opportunity to embrace aspects of the Chinese concept to conform to their own health infrastructure. WHO's "health for all" proclamation added impetus and encouragement to the new thinking – that primary health care can best serve the needs of resource-poor countries, because the concept is definitely cost-beneficial compared to the curative option, and, additionally, provides the exposure for extensive levels of contact between the health care providers and the community. Whether or not, the countries would use the "barefoot doctors" approach in like manner as China was immaterial. The lesson learnt was that auxiliary assistance could supplement the delivery of health services in poor countries, and could be a considerate option for some countries.

Like all transitions, health care priorities remain a challenge to this day in most countries, including many middle-income and developed countries. This dilemma continues to be a source of serious problems for the delivery of medical/public health services in about all the poor countries of the world. Evidence supports both the applicability and workability of primary health care principles as the option to benefit most people in need of care. Success will depend on "real collaboration" between government, the private sector, and donor organizations/countries, and the optimal use of resources to maximize benefits to the people served.

The real "fork in the road" for the future of global health progressivism is to accept the process of constant change and the important role of rationality and reasonableness in the formation of policy to transform the world's public health system into a meaningful program to meet current and future needs. This would involve a continued examination of the course to follow and the ability to modify objectives when problems arise. Global health policies would never be straightforward and the establishment of goals with long-term impact is fraught with uncertainty and the likelihood of failure, if not properly managed. Unfortunately, WHO in their quest to be looked at and considered a truly just institution, have unwittingly overlooked potential limitations to correct the challenging widespread and complex health problems globally in their efforts to create truly just societies throughout the world. That could be readily understood, but it is something that must be avoided in the future to maintain the utmost in credibility. We can still aspire together, and, doubtless, will achieve together, for the benefit of mankind's health, but not necessarily with goals that parallel "health for all" 2000, in spite of the rightness and idealism of the program, and the dreams of those who developed it.

"Reducing risks to health is the responsibility of governments – but not only of governments. It rightfully remains a vital of all people, in all populations, and of all those who serve them."
Gro Harlem Brundtland
WHO, Geneva, October 2002

"We have to ask ourselves whether medicine is to remain a humanitarian and respected profession or a new but science in the service of prolonging life rather than diminishing human suffering."
Elizabeth Kubler-Ross, 1926-

Chapter 3

The Millennium Development Goals: A Perspective

Historical Background/Introduction/Goals

The disappointing results of "Health for All 2000" provided impetus, and, one could logically concede was a major factor, if not the major factor, that forced the United Nations (UN) to conduct an intensive form of self-examination and overall assessment of the whys of what many global health advocates considered a program failure. While failure is a harsh conclusion and should be subjected to reasoned debate, and not mere condemnation, it is often overlooked in discourses of world health issues. This is so because many of the planned initiatives for health are longitudinal and overall responsibility and accountability is always retrospective, providing the opportunity for debate and analysis. Doubtless, those who were responsible for formatting "health for all 2000" over two decades ago meant well, based on conditions and circumstances at the time, and should not be subjected to an indictment or unnecessary criticism for the outcome. After all, they were gathered for the public good to serve what they perceived to be the challenges at the time and to promote a workable global health agenda to address the diverse needs of people throughout a complex world. Nonetheless, about twenty years later, a new holistic vision for global health care had to be re-visited, to bridge the gap, so to speak, if there was any hope to maintain some form of international momentum and improve on and accelerate some of the incomplete objectives established in "health for all 2000."

This was addressed in September 2000 at the United Nations Headquarters in New York when world leaders assembled once again to promote and adopt a new modified initiative – the United

Nations Millennium Declaration – committing all 192 UN member nations to eight well-defined goals with supporting descriptive targets and measurable indicators, deemed the Millennium Development Goals (MDGs). It is easy to fully understand the timeframe of the MDGs, since it is unusual and not in keeping with UN/WHO, World Bank, UNICEF, and other major actors in the field of global health, not to have an active, ongoing, and well-defined coordinated agenda for the promotion of world health as an organizational mission. It would be a departure from tradition; so, when the curtain came down on "health for all 2000," in the early fall of the same year, the MDGs became the new mantra and renewed vision for social development and health globally.

The goals and major targets are:

Goal 1: Eradicate extreme poverty and hunger

- Halve the proportion of people living on less than $1 a day
- Achieve decent employment for women, men, and young people
- Halve the proportion of people who suffer from hunger

Goal 2: Achieve universal primary education

- By 2015, all children can complete a full course of primary schooling, girls and boys

Goal 3: Promote gender equality and empower women

- Eliminate gender disparity in primary and secondary education preferably by 2005, and at all levels by 2015

Goal 4: Reduce child mortality

- Reduce by two-thirds, between 1990 and 2015, the under-five mortality rate

Goal 5: Improve maternal health

- Reduce by three quarters, between 1990 and 2015, the maternal mortality ratio
- Achieve, by 2015, universal access to reproductive health

Goal 6: Combat HIV/AIDS, malaria, and other diseases

- Have halted by 2015 and begun to reverse the spread of HIV/AIDS
- Achieve, by 2010, universal access to treatment for HIV/AIDS for all those who need it
- Have halted by 2015 and begun to reverse the incidence of malaria and other major diseases

Goal 7: Ensure environmental sustainability

- Integrate the principles of sustainable development into country policies and programs; reverse loss of environmental resources
- Reduce biodiversity loss, achieving, by 2010, a significant reduction in the rate of loss
- Halve, by 2015, the proportion of people without sustainable access to safe drinking water and basic sanitation
- By 2020, to have achieved a significant improvement in the lives of at least 100 million slum-dwellers

Goal 8: Develop a global partnership for development

- Develop further an open, rule-based, predictable, non-discriminatory trading and financial system
- Address the special needs of the least developed countries (LDC)
- Address the special needs of landlocked countries and small island developing States
- Deal comprehensively with the debt problem of developing countries through national and international measures in order to make debt sustainable in the long term
- In co-operation with pharmaceutical companies, provide access to affordable, essential drugs in developing countries
- In co-operation with the private sector, make available the benefits of new technologies, especially information and communications

The Pertinence of the Millennium Development
Goals (MDGs) to Global Health

The advent of 2000 witnessed the world's health planners and decision makers examining many of the existing deficiencies that were, hopefully, to be achieved by a successful "health for all 2000" initiative proposed in 1978. That existing and demanding conundrum forced an acute response by the United Nations to ascertain that some type of formal momentum had to be developed in a timely manner to replace the vacuum left by "health for all 2000" to address the continuing challenges still faced by global health at the turn of the century. The dreams of the Alma Ata assembly that gave the world "health for all 2000" by instituting primary health care correctives about two decades earlier had distinct shortfalls, some critics claimed failure, even using the most reasonable evaluative criteria of outcome assessment. Renewed dimensions of global health reform, therefore, had to be re-examined with immediacy to fill the void, and that, not surprisingly, took the form of another declaration with a new set of exciting and ambitious goals, the Millennium Development Goals (MDGs) in the year 2000. Targets to the goals were descriptive and were added in 2001 as supplements to assist countries as operational guidelines to achieve the objectives, particularly the less developed countries with a paucity of human resources, and limited infrastructures for planning and organizational management.

The philosophy of the new MDGs was the pursuance of a more concerted and aggressive approach that heightened with priorities many dimensions of national development with emphasis on social and economic improvements in the less developed countries. That creates a compelling challenge because there is no wonderful magic formula that will be just right to address the diversity of complex issues facing public health and social reform in the least developed countries, and for that matter, just about all countries. The structuring and organization of public health programs have traditionally been ad hoc and lacking in long-term commitment and

46

sustainability, contributing to unsatisfactory outcomes and disappointments, and the resulting reactive sentiments of a large cohort of public health advocates, at both the national and global levels, who have developed serious doubts and reservations about declarations, period! This is most unfortunate, because so many poor countries lack elementary capabilities and have needs that are so compelling that we should never forget our commitment, as a global brotherhood, to work collaboratively to promote the benefits of common values that will help create a compassionate world that will eliminate misery, malnutrition/hunger, unnecessary morbidity and mortality, and the general deprivation of so many people in a world of plenty. Pessimism is not prescriptive, and while evidence in many countries give reason for it, we have to continue with resolve and tenacity to succeed.

There is, also, sadly, no operational measure that decision makers can resort to or agree on to meet needs across the board globally for countries. Additionally, while social and economic improvements are all embracing terms that are generally acceptable by health planners in government and politicians, they are fraught with ambiguity and defy a reliable measure for assessment, because of a lack of specificity and vagueness. It would seem more appropriate to consider some basic primary goals regionally, for example, select countries of sub-Saharan Africa and South Asia could be used as bases to promote the introduction of fundamental human rights, including something as elementary as the right to clean water, improvement of health care services at rural clinics, and compulsory childhood education as worthy objectives based on financial capabilities and in conformance with the needs of the population and political direction of individual countries. This approach will seem most applicable and amplifies the one step at a time philosophy that could meet the needs of many of the less developed countries that lack resources for governance intra and inter-agencies. Granted, that aspects/concepts of the aforementioned are within the MDGs, but the comprehensiveness of the goals would overwhelm the resource capabilities of many of the poor countries.

Progressivism of the current Millennium Development Goals (MDGs) is still totally dependent and linked to the sustainability of the economic status of countries. This deficit, like others, is most applicable to developing countries. That will continue to remain a challenging dichotomy and a distinct paradox, as attempts to move to the next tier by reforming health care in emerging economies are programmed. Countries can never experience upward mobility in health care or other forms of social progression and opportunities with the hope for improved standards of living and equity when populations are burdened by a continuum of health and environmental hazards, poverty – extreme in many countries, excess morbidity and mortality, and a lack of financial resources and infrastructures to build on governance and services. It is more practical to consider the benefits that accrue from narrowly focused programs to build on public goods and needs than spreading resources thin on many different fronts. So, while the need for MDGs is not a part of the debate because of its rationality and obviously clear applicability that will substantially benefit the lives of the poor in developing countries, the goals, nonetheless, have to be tempered in such a way that progress and ultimate success can be the outcome, and not just another customary declaration of broad and disparate goals with a potential for failure.

The MDGs, like "health for all 2000" present an affront and dilemma to many developing countries that lack the constructs, know-how, and paucity of resources to truly make the goals a success. That should not be viewed as symptomatic of indifference, but the reality of the lack of existing capability in poor countries, even when the benefits of most objectives are apparent and appreciated. Global health strategists, therefore, should learn from history and prevent the perpetuation of long-term programs in a world of never-ending uncertainty, and little hope of sustainability for successful health outcomes. A failure to learn from history also guarantees the repetition of ill-conceived ideologies for global health in a world that badly needs health reforms and the interventions of public health practice to serve billions of people who remain at risk and vulnerable.

The Challenges for Achieving the Goals by 2015

There is no surprise of the results of the interim assessments measuring the progress of countries in the achievement of the MDGs within the established timeframes. Interestingly, two major countries of interest, China and India, with approximately one third of the world's population, have shown marked improvements in poverty reduction due predominantly to economic growth and development in both countries. Without being trite, these countries have definite ambitions in proving that they are now major forces on the world's stage economically, and take pride in demonstrating their commitments to sustainable development from the broadest meaning of the word, including health care reform, and overall improvements and modernization of their social welfare and public health programs.

China's continuing economic surges defy a logical explanation. They were not only spectacular, but exceeded expectations, leaving many economists and development experts in the Western world to wonder and ponder of the country's impressive accomplishments. India, on the other hand, although lacking the surprise and dramatic economic performance of China, nonetheless, started its own recovery through needed reforms and has made inroads to combat the chronic depressing state of poverty that has challenged the country's political leadership for decades. While both countries are still burdened by serious pressing problems of every conceivable perspective, varying from environmental degradation to a continuing and embarrassing inequity, the energy and momentum in both countries provide cause for hope that poverty alleviation, improved health care for the masses, and the other major goals of universal primary education, gender inequity, including the utility of global partnerships, while still formidable challenges, can be viewed with greater optimism than at any time in the history of the two countries.

Obviously, this trend is important for the progressivism of the MDGs. In fact, we are dealing with one third of humanity, and this could be the necessary exemplar for other developing countries to emulate, especially considering the hurdles that both countries faced in arriving at their destination of better tomorrows for their people. That does not signify in any way celebratory closure that the end of poverty and its antecedents and associated misery have disappeared, but, it does mean that both countries, with a sense of pride and determination, have instituted correctives to ascertain that their people will enjoy a better standard of living based on a renewed agenda for social and economic development.

This book will make no attempt to examine poverty from all the different constructs of income, consumption, minimal needs for sustenance or relative deprivation. The subject is replete with references that address the varied nuances of poverty and the ripple effect on people, especially in the less developed countries of the world. It would use nothing more than the crude macro-assessment of the subject – when you see it, you automatically recognize it. On visits to the least developed countries, no one has to describe or define poverty. It is totally apparent and leaves its mark on all who are truly attuned to the elements of social justice. I am reminded of a judge in one of the courts providing an opinion on pornography or what is pornographic material who wisely opined, I will recognize it when I see it. The same principle applies to poverty. The manifestations, much like pornography cannot hide. They are fully transparent.

Not surprisingly, the region of the world needing the benefits of the MDGs' stimulus the most, sub-Saharan Africa, have not witnessed any dramatic changes in their quality of life or living standards. Some countries have actually lost ground, so to speak, instead of making progress. The overall results are definitely not encouraging. This basically means that unless draconian efforts are instituted immediately, the countries of this region, and many other poor countries, extern to sub-Saharan Africa, for example, parts of Asia, Latin America, and the Caribbean, the defined goals and targets would not be achieved. This could result in a catastrophic defeat to global public health and would further undermine the credibility of the organizations that promote these holistic all-embracing, and uplifting ambitious goals.

A strong current of negativity and doubt has started to emerge as analyses of the MDGs demonstrate serious problems being faced by many countries. The Institute of Development Studies (IDS) in a policy brief in June 2009 began to highlight the existing global economic uncertainties and the likely necessity to evaluate the worthiness and workability of the MDG concept for global development. Predictably, the question surfaced whether or not another type of system is an option if the MDGs are not realized. On a personal note, while we must never lack optimism when it comes to the welfare and health of people, the thought of another failed initiative should be cause for a thorough examination of the possibility of another failure. This is the epitome of humiliation. Why? Examine the record – the Universal Declaration of Human

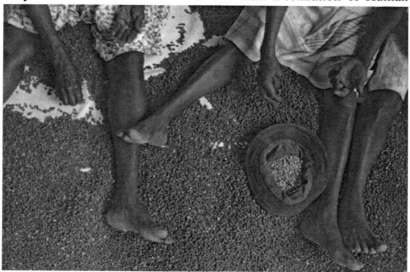

Rights, Health for All by the Year 2000, now the Millennium Development Goals!!!

The mere approach to the MDGs by the establishment of fixed and defined goals seems flawed in many ways, and supporting evidence from some countries affirms this concern. The goals were meant as global targets, but measurements and assessments were at a national level challenging the basics of uniformity and distorting the true picture for putting together a realistic status quo during interim evaluations. Additionally, many developing countries had serious reservations about the applicability and what to them seemed an inappropriate imposition of targets that did not reflect the wishes or needs of the local population. An example is the subject of continuing conflict and internal strife in many countries inhabited by nearly one third of the world's poorest people, and having a severe impact on stability and development. This, unfortunately, has resulted in no progress in the reduction of extreme poverty and maternal mortality contributing in many cases to conditions that have become more acute and worse in some countries. The MDGs, should they fail, will perpetuate the continuum of millions of preventable diseases and premature deaths, and could make the future for development aid and assistance for the world's most vulnerable and poor people more challenging and difficult in the future.

Eradicate Extreme Poverty and Hunger

Extreme poverty is a condition of bare survival, beneath any human decency and with very limited hope, affecting one fifth of the world's population. Poverty and hunger is as old as humanity, and an integral part of the history of mankind. The Bible described varied issues of the plight of the poor and the hungry. For centuries, there have been efforts and strategic plans globally to marginalize world hunger and alleviate the blight of poverty, the precursor of hunger. World hunger is a symptom of world poverty, and distressingly challenging, because of the ubiquitous nature of the problem in poor and underdeveloped countries. The targets to halve the proportion of people living on less than $1 a day; achieve decent employment for women, men, and young people; and halve the proportion of people who suffer from hunger by 2015, while a mixture of humanitarian

52

idealism and social justice, and, the right thing to do, sadly would never be realized within the timeframe.

The commitment, financial support, and the will needed to improve the lives of those affected by extreme poverty (those living on less than $1 a day), no or under employment, and the continuing widespread hunger and inequality in most developing countries is nothing short of herculean. Sadly, outside of China, poverty in developing countries has increased over the last 25 years, and, not surprisingly, the worst failure is in Africa where the number of people living in extreme poverty has doubled. The intent of the goal to eradicate extreme poverty and hunger is humane, uplifting, and the absolutely proper response of governments and the global public health community. But, examined from a broad range of determinants, the goal based on current and future parameters is hyper-optimistic and will not be achieved.

This is another example in global policy intervention where the most ambitious and worthy causes have to face the indignity and pain of reality and failure. Life for the poor of the world remains a brutal experience, much like living in bondage, and awaiting freedom! Add to this some indicators that in many of the developing countries, extreme poverty and hunger have gotten worse, and not limited to Africa, although this continent continues to be the epicenter of destitution. These conditions approximate a sense of hopelessness, and remain an international disgrace, and a mandate for new solutions and a renewed resolve for correctives. Finding the most expeditious way remains the challenge. The problem is, can we find a way.

Achieve Universal Primary Education

For decades, the goal for achieving universal primary education has been discussed as an ideal. Educators and governments throughout the world have recognized the potential benefits of varied aspects and concepts of education as a window for development that could enhance economic growth and social well-being. During international symposia, advocates from throughout the world have defined and agreed in principle how universal primary education could be a resource for alleviating poverty, enhance the improvement of living and health standards, particularly in developing countries, and become an empowerment tool to promote literacy. The MDG second goal has specifically targeted that all children, regardless of gender, can complete a full course of primary schooling by 2015.

According to the World Bank in 2004, more than 100 million primary school age children remain out of school, despite the promise since 1990 that all children would be able to complete a full course of primary education. Realistically, if there is the slightest semblance of hope for this goal to be achieved by 2015, school systems in all developing countries "will need to train teachers, build classrooms, and improve the quality of education. Most important, they will have to remove such barriers to attendance as fees and lack of transportation, and address parents concern for the safety of their children." Six years later, Ashley Seager of the Guardian (United Kingdom) reported on January 20, 2010, on the severe negative consequences that the global recession was having on any hope for progress of universal primary education. The article further illuminated that the initiative is "being knocked off course by the global financial crisis, which is leaving a legacy of rising poverty and hunger." The obvious result is that socially-marginalized children in nearly all developing countries, particularly in sub-Saharan Africa, will continue to suffer the indignity of educational inequality, and a future that will suppress any chance for a better standard of living, and, indeed, hope for the future.

In 2007, a privately funded study by the American Academy of Arts and Sciences confirms cause for pessimism. While there were semblances of overall improvements globally, long term estimates determined that about one in six children of primary school age, or about 114 million, would not be enrolled in 2015. These estimates could be considered the best-case scenario, typical of reports of this nature in the consideration of the inconsistencies in assembling and authenticating data. While primary education was amplified in the study, the same research also indicated that about 185 million children, approximately one in four, will not be attending secondary schools by the year 2015. Unfortunately, strategic investments in education to build good national institutions and assure access to good educational quality would not be realized in most, if not all of the less developed countries. This situation applies especially to countries of sub-Saharan Africa, Asia, some countries in the Middle East, Latin America, and the Caribbean. Signs of encouragement in many countries are nothing more than what needs to be done, and in no way approximate any significant educational sustainability that will contribute to development. Nonetheless, it is a positive factor in improving infrastructure within a country. Each country's educational policy and programs are important indicators of not only how well it is doing in the broad sphere of advancing education, but also as a mechanism for providing the citizenry a way up and out of poverty by enhancing opportunities for better jobs through education while building on intellectual capital that could contribute to sustained economic stabilization within communities and a nation as a whole. Education opens up minds and assists in confidence building and hope, important ingredients for developing countries as forces for social and economic momentum and change.

Promote Gender Equality and Empower Women
The promotion of gender equality and the empowerment of women through the elimination of disparities in primary and secondary education by 2005, and at all levels by 2015 is another noble goal that would have to remain a moral imperative, because it will not be accomplished during the defined timeframe, despite the various forms of gender injustice that limits and marginalizes women's rights and educational opportunities for growth. There is evidence, however, that while some improvements have taken place at the primary level, gender disparities remain a compelling affront to educators in most developing countries. This lack of "upward mobility" and progress hinders the benefits that could be derived from universal primary education as a construct for modeling a

country's knowledge and training base that is vitally needed to compete and succeed in society and could also ultimately contribute to the alleviation of poverty and hunger, and the formatting of disease control and prevention infrastructures, leading to well-being and a better standard of living for people. The ideal remains overall sustainable development at all national levels to enhance opportunities that will permit girls and women to gain footing on the social ladder of success.

On the primary and secondary school enrollment challenge, a United Nations report did not offer any encouraging insights or optimism for the future. The findings were dire and illustrated that of the 113 countries that failed the 2005 objective, only 18 of those countries are likely to meet the goal by 2015. The out of school population, not surprisingly, comprised 55 percent of girls. Without 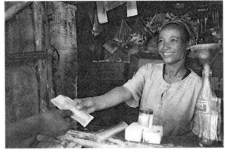 a basic education that will provide an introduction to learning the fundamentals of reading and writing, the ultimate goal of building on a foundation to empower women to achieve their developmental potential in a sustainable manner has no footing and mocks UNICEF's definition of the hope of "leveling the playing field for girls and women.....to develop their talents."

Gender biases deny women their basic rights in many societies throughout the world, something as elemental as the right to own land and property in some countries, full and decent employment with equitable treatment, and opportunities to participate in business ventures by gaining access to funding, that would normally go to men, especially in rural regions. This lack of access and discrimination to land and credit, and the meaningful pursuit of economic initiatives are limited due to traditions and sometimes religious and legal constraints. Change, however, has started to emerge slowly, and the windows of opportunity have began to open, albeit, slowly.

Early marriages of mostly uneducated girls contribute to alarming rates of maternal morbidity and mortality. Annually, using a conservative estimate, over 500,000 women die giving birth, and, not surprisingly, like all the other cumulative challenges, ninety-nine percent of the deaths occur in developing countries. Violence against women remains a problem and a continuing source of injustice in many societies, contributing to the broad range of disparities that marginalize females in general, some caused by complex social, religious, and cultural facets that will take time and understanding for both the institution of change, and the reality of change.

Reduce Child Mortality

Maternal mortality, neonatal mortality (the number of children dying under the age of 28 days), infant mortality (death under 1 year old), and child mortality (deaths of children under the age of five) have been used as determinants and indicators of national health programs for decades, and, from a more inclusive perspective for centuries, to a limited degree. The child mortality criterion has become the accepted standard for global assessments, providing comparative and reasoned insights of how individual countries are performing in this category. Caution is, however, in order, and we must accede and accept that regardless of the best of efforts made by all institutions at data collection of vital statistics in developing countries, deficits in many national systems could skew the data and influence findings and results. Nonetheless, accepting the premise that dealing with data at a global level is never simple or easy, we present some of the latest peer review published findings to heighten the MDG 4, to reduce by two-thirds the under the age of five mortality rate between 1990 and 2015, and the other inferences of the goal.

Recapitulating briefly that there are always limits to analyses using numbers, and the pertinence and interpretation of findings, we have selected references provided by reputable organizations, regardless of the potential imperfections of numbers, based on peer review and what has historically been accepted worldwide. We understand the analogy that we do not live in a perfect world, and that study findings could find varying interpretations; so, like all other facets of epidemiology, we plead for understanding.

Researchers from the University of Washington (Seattle), using what they considered to be a more complete and accurate calculation than previously used, determined that the deaths of children under the age of five has decreased in the last two decades (1990-2010) from 11.9 million in 1990 to 7.7 million in 2010. The lead researcher in the study indicated that the decision to double the amount of data evaluated improved and refined the estimation and assisted in the conclusion that in general children are doing better today, mortality wise, than at any time in recent history. While this statement is general and could be subject to debate, it, however, illustrates reason for guarded optimism.

Interestingly, the University of Washington research findings closely approximated research done by UNICEF (September 2009 report) that suggested the improved results could be attributed to better techniques for the prevention of malaria, and a more efficient use of drugs to assist babies born to mothers infected with the HIV/AIDS virus, both major causes of child mortality in poor countries. The UNICEF report showed that the child mortality rate declined by more than a quarter, from 90 per 1,000 in 1990, to 65 per 1,000 in 2009. An additional inference relating to these numbers is that there are 10,000 less child deaths daily throughout the world. This should be cause for elation!

Many of the most unanticipated and impressive achievements in the past two decades came from countries that historically had the highest rate of child mortality. Ethiopia is a case in point that amplifies the success enjoyed by some countries – the country's child mortality rate had dropped by half during the period of 1990 to 2010. An interesting comparative finding is that Singapore, a small progressive Asian "giant," in its own right, has the lowest under five mortality rate in the world, equating to 2 deaths per 1,000. The

United States, in contrast, ranks 42nd in the world, with a child mortality rate of 6.7 per 1,000.

What we are witnessing based on the current findings is that fewer children under the five age category are dying around the world, particularly in the less developed countries where 99 percent of these, mostly avoidable deaths occur. The mortality comparatives remain markedly inequitable with about 50 percent of all deaths occurring in sub-Saharan Africa and 32 percent in South Asia, contributing to a depressing 82 percent of all child mortalities globally.

The constant challenge of child mortality remains. If there is any hope of achieving any success in child mortality globally, the rate would have to reach around a 4.4 percent reduction to meet the MDG 4 of two-thirds reduction of child mortality between 1990 and 2015. Sadly, sixty-seven of the countries considered high child mortality remain a serious and compelling challenge to global public health, and only about 10 of these countries, optimistically, have any realistic chance of achieving the reduction goal of MDG 4. And, the health of the public in many developing countries continues to be vulnerable and at risk to widespread poverty, hunger, and disease that serve as pathologics to development and the provision of equitable services, exemplified by the high prevalence of child mortality.

Improve Maternal Mortality

The maternal mortality rate is the number of maternal deaths per 100,000 live births, and is basically a reflection of the number of maternal deaths in a population associated with pregnancy or direct obstetric causes. The World Health Organization (WHO) in 1992 offered the following definition: "The death of a woman while pregnant or within 42 days of termination of pregnancy, irrespective of the duration and site of the pregnancy, from any cause related to or aggravated by the3 pregnancy or its management but not from accidental or incidental causes." Goal 5 of the MDGs specifically proposes to reduce by three-quarters, the maternal mortality ratio, between 1990 and 2015, and achieve, by the year 2015, universal access to reproductive health. Achieving goal 5 would require an annual decline of 5.5% in maternal mortality ratios between the period 1990 and 2015, and the current rate of progress provides no hope that the reduction would be realized. At the global level, assessments show maternal mortality has decreases at an average of less than 1% annually between 1990 and 2005, far below the necessary 5.5% decline to achieve MDG 5. The countries that have traditionally had the highest incidence of maternal mortality, the poorest countries, have made no appreciable progress over the past 15 years, and realistically, that trend will likely continue. Ninety-nine percent of all maternal deaths occur in developing countries, where the lifetime risk of death due to pregnancy and childbirth is 1 in 76, and a compelling mandate for improvement. That should be a defying and challenging statistic for global health strategists. The comparative for developed countries averages 1 in 8,000, with the risk in the United States being about 1 in 4,800. This continuing disparity is not only limited to rich and poor countries, but differences exist in urban compared to rural areas within countries, and women who are educated and those with no formal education. Unfortunately, the objective for any truly functional system of universal access to reproductive health in most developing countries, while a moral imperative based on needs, would not come close to achievement in most of the poor countries, especially problematic in regions of Africa and South Asia.

True and measured progress can be achieved by access to health care before (pre-natal), during, and after childbirth, skilled professional attendance at birth deliveries including the accessibility to hospital and midwifery care, control of infectious diseases and the complications linked to childbirth, education and upgrading of hospital and clinic staff with enhanced specialty training, and when feasible development of facility-based obstetric care, and generating national political support for women's rights.

The New York Times, reporting on results (April 15, 2010) based on a comprehensive study published in the prestigious medical journal, the Lancet, described that for the first time in decades the global mortality rate for maternal deaths declined from around 526,300 in 1980 to about 342,900 in 2008. This longitudinal study was funded by the Bill and Melinda Gates Foundation, an organization fully committed and attuned to improving global health, especially in resource-poor countries. Additionally, it provides a sense of the immense positive impact this foundation has in reforming the world's global health agenda.

All current determinants and indicators are that MDG 5 to improve maternal mortality, like just about all of the other seven goals, would not be achieved by 2015. In fact, only 12 percent of countries are expected to meet the goal. Pregnancy and childbirth, the epicenter of womanhood, remain the leading causes of death in poor countries globally; one woman per minute dies while giving birth or soon after every day, and between 10-15 million annually in developing countries suffer serious injuries and complications in the act of giving birth. The thought, however, that foundations like Bill and Melinda Gates are involved to help conquer the inequitable ravages of maternal mortality affecting women in the developing countries provides every reason for hope and optimism, and serves as an impetus for all who are dedicated to the field of global health practice with intent to help the vulnerable majority who continue to remain at risk for every conceivable threat to health and well-being.

Combat HIV/AIDS, Malaria, and Other Diseases
The MDG 6 is geared towards halting and reversing the spread of HIV/AIDS by 2015, achieving by 2010, universal access to treatment for HIV/AIDS for all who need it, and halting and reversing the incidence of malaria and other major diseases (like tuberculosis) by 2015, as the major targets. While the specific highlighted diseases of the goal are HIV/AIDS and malaria, many international initiatives have identified tuberculosis as a logical disease for inclusion. Thus, while these three major diseases would be amplified under MDG 6, the challenging impact and influence of the plethora of other diseases that continue to threaten the poor

countries of the world cannot be overlooked, and would be addressed in other segments of the book. The validation for heightening is that these three diseases remain thematic with all international organizations as urgent and in need of special emphasis recognition because of the health and social debilitation impact that they have had and continue to have on so many poor countries, in every sector of the world. In fact, the three diseases have been dubbed by many in the academic and public health community, including the World Health Organization, as diseases of poverty and in need of prioritizing immediacy.

The global population today is estimated to be approximately 6,706,993,152. Of this population, reasoned estimates (likely conservative, nonetheless) are that 32,900,000 are infected with the HIV/AIDS virus, 13,722,534 are suffering from tuberculosis, and there are about 247,000,000 cases of malaria. Additionally, the mortality perspective indicates that annually on an average, HIV/AIDS kills about 2.1 million people, 1.7 million die from tuberculosis, and malaria kills about 1 million. These diseases disproportionately and consistently affect the poorest of the planet, and Africa, the continent that continues to be of major concern to global health planners, remains the most impacted by the cumulative effect of these three diseases that kill an average of over 8,500 people on the continent daily.

HIV/AIDS is on the verge of wiping out a whole generation during their most precious and productive years of life, and over 12 million children in Africa have suffered the loss of one or both parents to the disease, creating pockets of a socio-economic crisis in many countries on the continent. While the cost for antiretroviral medicines have decreased substantially, providing a greater opportunity for treatment for many of the infected, the cycle of transmission of the disease remains a distinct affront – 7,000 people are infected with the virus daily. The move forward to meaningful prevention and control continues on a tenuous track full of obstacles and barriers.

Estimated prevalence (the number of HIV/AIDS cases as a percentage of the population aged 15 to 49 years) is used to monitor the world's HIV/AIDS epidemic. Annually, about 3.1 million people die of AIDS, with approximately 500,000 being children under the age of 15. The worst affected remain inhabitants of sub-Saharan Africa where prevalence rates in countries of the region vary from 7.2 to 30 percent. Prevention is paramount in assuring disease control and prevention through education, since there is no cure for the disease. Unfortunately, millions continue to live in darkness and know very little about the transmission of the disease and how to protect themselves against the infectious onslaught of the virus. This situation persists, in spite of concerted efforts by public health authorities in many countries of the developing world to get the message of HIV/AIDS prevention to populations at risk. Hope for prevention of HIV is centered in the discovery and availability of an effective vaccine. Until this is realized, the traditional prevention methods of safe sex and the avoidance of injection-drug use, and sharing of needles remain highly recommended.

Retrospectively, there is a semblance of utmost irony when we consider that at the dawn of the 21st century, we are still suggesting immediacy and priority for the control and prevention of a disease like tuberculosis that has been described in humans since antiquity, going back to tubercular lesions observed in Egyptian mummies around 2400 B.C. Just as pertinent, and historically fascinating and informative, is that malaria, one of the oldest diseases of mankind has linkages that can be traced to clay tablets written several thousand years ago.

Malaria is an integral part of the annals of medicine, having been described in early Chinese and Indian writings more than 3,000 years ago. The disease is endemic in at least ninety-one countries, putting about 40% of the world's population at risk. WHO reports the global incidence of the disease between 300,000,000 to 500,000,000, causing between 1,500,000 to 2,700,000 deaths. This makes malaria one of the greatest causes of morbidity and mortality in the world today, with increased risk for pregnant women and children under the age of five.

Tuberculosis, a disease that many infectious disease experts thought potentially controllable, has re-emerged as a major defiant threat to global public health. Prevalence trends in the last decade continue to increase, killing about 1,700,000 annually. About 230,000 of the deaths are linked to concomitant HIV infection. About 99% of the infected/affected live in the developing countries of Africa and Asia, validating the constant challenge to health in the resource-poor regions of the world. Like just about all other factors associated with risk, the poor in all developing countries remain the most vulnerable, compounded by the effects of malnutrition, which compromises the immune system, and lack of proper treatment. Like other diseases of poverty, most of the deaths occur during the most productive years of life, between the ages of fifteen and fifty-four.

At the G8 conference in Okinawa, Japan, January 2000, it was consensual that a greater effort was needed to combat HIV/AIDS, malaria, and tuberculosis. This recognition contributed to the founding of the Global Fund in 2002 in Geneva, Switzerland, with the compelling objective to:

"Attract, manage and disburse additional resources through a new public-private partnership that will make a sustainable and significant contribution to the reduction of infections, illnesses, and deaths, thereby mitigating the impact caused by HIV/AIDS, tuberculosis, and malaria in countries in need and contributing to poverty reduction as part of the Millennium Development goals."

Analytically, there is no evidence or indicators of any hope for the achievement of this goal. In fact, risk determinants by infectious disease epidemiologists show signs that some countries would actually experience an increased risk from certain aspects of these three referenced diseases than existed when the goal was first established in 2000. This is exemplary of how making futuristic projections for disease goals through control and prevention globally could be so complex, frustrating, uncertain, and, most often, disappointing – regardless of how moral and noble those goals may be.

Ensure Environmental Sustainability

Goal 7 of the MDGs, ensure environmental sustainability, targets and highlights as themes for achievement, the integration of the principle of sustainable development into country policies and programs and reversing the loss of environmental resources; reducing biodiversity loss, and, achieving by 2010, a significant reduction in the rate of loss; halving by 2015, the proportion of people without sustainable access to safe drinking water and basic sanitation; and by 2020, to have achieved a significant improvement in the lives of at least 100 million slum dwellers.

During the last three decades, concerns of the environment globally have been heightened and have become the focus of serious attention by national and international organizations, including many in leadership roles in developing countries where environmental degradation is seen as a challenging deterrent to growth and development, and the hope of economic stability. The wanton abuse of land, and the resources of the land, air and water pollution, the accumulation of greenhouse gases, lack of a governing advocacy for the environment, fragile infrastructure, and global warning, support the rising anxiety that if environmental assault is not curtailed, the quality of life and human well-being in general will be endangered, especially in the resource-poor countries, already burdened by all forms of endangerment. Environmental sustainability ("meeting current human needs without undermining the capacity of the environment to provide for these needs over the long term") has been proposed as the mantra for reform and its pertinence magnified by the U.N. Millennium Declaration that stated we must "spare no effort to free all of humanity, and above all our children and grandchildren, from the threat of living on a planet irredeemably spoilt by human activities, and whose resources would no longer be sufficient for their needs."

The situation and conditions today, in spite of our best intentions to institute meaningful changes to make the lives of people better, through improved modifications of the environment, remain appalling. Throughout our planet, nearly 15 percent of the population (a conservative estimate), lack clean drinking water. In some of the poorest countries, there are no reliable estimates, and consensus is that those numbers could be much higher, especially in the rural areas, where water becomes a luxury for many, and the percentages of those who are able to assess it approximate 50 percent. Over 35 percent or 2.4 billion people lack any access to sanitary/hygienic facilities, and 20 percent or 1.2 billion people have no link to basic sanitation facilities. The aforementioned amplifies dramatically the serious gaps that exist between developed and developing countries in the fundamentals that contribute to the practice and policies of public health, and the concurrent impact of the continuing deficits that overwhelmingly affect the disadvantaged poor living in poverty

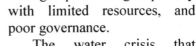

with limited resources, and poor governance.

The water crisis that continues as a deterrent in most developing countries to this day prevents initiatives to build on biodiversity that has the potential to enhance a sustainable ecosystem that would assist economic growth, development, stability, and ultimately human welfare. For example, there is no hope to develop and build on natural ecosystems for food production, and other venture objectives without water, even though many developing countries, by nature, traditions, and practices, could adapt readily at transforming their ecosystems for long-term productivity and growth. I mention food, because it is integral to life and survival in all countries, but has special relevance to developing countries, because of occasional scarcities. This has an overall tremendous negative influence on the socio-economic problems faced by the rural poor in most developing countries. The option often resorted to is migration to urban settings to look for jobs away from home, disrupting family lives, and contributing to slum-dwelling, and the social challenges and problems associated with that form of marginal existence, paralleling little more than getting by barely, one day at a time, with few dreams, other than being able to go home to see family, again, if possible.

The promotion, progress, and success of the collective efforts to improve environmental sustainability will obviously play an important and significant role in helping to alleviate poverty, hunger, and disease, and would enhance the quality of life and improve standards of living and health of populations in developing countries. Sadly, however, in many poor countries, it is impossible to determine where the slum begins or ends. There seems to be no apparent boundaries, just one big form of interconnectedness of slum dwelling. In some of the overcrowded cities of Africa, Asia, and some of the less developed countries, slum dwelling, disappointingly, has become the only thing known by generations of people for decades, without a vista for change, and that cycle perpetuates itself, too often.

A reasoned analysis of the current global status for MDG 7 and the noble objectives and targets associated with it, provide little assurance that the goal has any hope of being achieved, at least within the established timeframe. We can celebrate the intent and goodness of the goal. We recognize that there continue to be signs of improvement in varied spheres of the environmental movement towards some semblances of sustainability in many resource-poor countries, including the utmost dedication of so many devotees, who are motivated to make the world an improved place for all to cherish and enjoy, environmentally and otherwise. Nevertheless, reality pains. There is so much more that has to be done, and the future continues to be as doubtful today as when the global health/social advocates advanced the original idea of the broad benefits of environmental sustainability with the hope of instituting reform, particularly for the less developed countries of the globe.

Develop a Global Partnership for Development

MDG 8, plans to develop a global partnership for development with defined and specific targets for an open, rule-based, predictable non-discriminatory trading and financial system; address the special needs of the least developed countries (LDCs), landlocked developing countries and small island developing States; dealing with the debt problems of developing countries; co-operating with pharmaceutical companies for improved access to essential drugs in poor countries; and collaboration with the private sector to increase the availability of new technologies, like information and communication.

According to a United Nations report on the progress of MDG 8, official development assistance (ODA) from donor countries continues to drop due to a decrease in debt relief grants, decline in exchange rates, and adjusting for changes in prices of commodities and goods. Developed countries will have to increase donations, some markedly so, over the next few years, to compensate for the financial commitments made in 2005 to assist resource-poor countries. This hoped for and much anticipated increase in financial aid will likely not occur due to the global economic downturn being experienced by donor countries that traditionally support development programs. While developed countries have been involved in the major aspects of hastening growth and development, debt relief, fair trade and equitable practices, and direct investment in many ventures in the emerging economies of developing countries, an important trust of the goal is for developing countries themselves to create the momentum to achieve steady and continuous economic growth and sustainability within their borders. These targets have been slowed to a standstill due to the uncertainty and turmoil taking place in the global economy. The obvious is when donors are in financial trouble, clouded by a series of unknowns, recipients suffer. It is a predictable and understood cycle. If there are any doubts or reservations of the current trend, a recent report from the United States would affirm the economic relevance. Donations to organizations and causes in 2009 were 303 billion dollars, the lowest amount since 1956. The acuteness of the trend is real. The concern is that it could continue longer due to the crises in different sectors of the globe.

Open and non-discriminatory trade liberalization was the mantra for prosperity at the end of the 20th century and the start of the 21st. The logic was that developed countries would open doors and opportunities/options for exports from developing countries, and make the concept of globalization work their magnificent wonders as envisioned by proponents. This worldwide form of open trade initiative and "dream" to level the playing field, so to speak, has improved slightly, depending to whom you listen, but nowhere near the potential anticipated by MDG 8. A disappointing and uncontrollable aspect of trade is that even if the process was truly liberalized and equitable, not all countries could enjoy the benefits, nor share in the possible economic upturn, because many developing countries, despite yeoman efforts in recent years, are unable to conform to the quality and safety standards of importing countries of the developed world, thus perpetuating inequity that must be corrective for free and fair trade to work.

The special needs of the least developed countries will persist as a compelling charge, and while there have been evidence of small successes in some countries, collectively, the future is stacked with problems that have to be overcome if there is any hope for moving forward without generous assistance from donor countries or organizations. The cancellation of a country's debts is great; but, that is not what the future is all about. The road to self-sufficiency should be a foremost priority for the least developed countries, or at least a goal to the continuous improvement of economic development, good governance, poverty reduction and hopefully an improved standard of living, devoid of dependency for everyone and everything. A distinct degree of commonality, albeit, from different perspectives, apply also to the landlocked developing countries and small island States in transition, and reason for serious assessment also, because of the myriad challenges these countries face. These conditions and circumstances, cumulatively, will remain a defying affront to development economists, sociologists, and health strategists, for many years in the future, who are intent on being involved with transformations for sustained improvements in these countries. Dependency will continue to limit freedom and the ability for development, free from the control or influence of others in many countries. That is not, however, what the developing countries need in perpetuity. Granted, true freedom and independence will take decades for some countries to fully enjoy, but, nonetheless, they should remain a central focus to progress, self-sufficiency and economic momentum.

Discussion

Longitudinal worldwide goals, regardless of what form they take, or what they objectify, whether economic, general development and growth, social or health, are always fraught with unknowns and potentially unanticipated outcomes, due to uncertainty and the inability to forecast across the planet, consisting of about 200 countries, and over 6 billion people with varied traditions, customs, religions, and cultures. The goals/objectives tend to become especially burdensome and limiting when the paramount anticipated result is to contribute to meaningful changes in improving the quality of life by alleviating ubiquitous poverty that impacts, in one form or another, about half of the globe's population, approximating over 3 billion people. Additionally, the generic characteristics of the MDGs, considered guideposts, apply equally across the broad spectrum of countries that possess clear and distinct differences. This is overwhelming. Even countries within a continent like Africa, the epicenter for the success of the "movement" like Benin, Mali, and

Malawi, are totally different from South Africa and Botswana. It is the same continent, different people, different problems, different history, and different culture and economic needs for growth and development to improve the lives of the people. We need a more individualistic or regional approach based on reasoned assessments by approaching the challenges in small bits at a time that would permit resource-poor infrastructures the opportunity for involvement and buy-in, instead of being told what to do. The sheer "bigness" of some of the goals becomes a burden for managers in poor countries. The same analogy applies to parts of Asia, Eastern Europe, and Latin America.

This analogy applies fully to a program like the Millennium Development Goals (MDGs), with broad, extensive, and diversified objectives and targets to institute changes, delving into spheres of poverty reduction, education, gender inequality, child and maternal mortality and health, disease prevention and control, advocacy for environmental sustainability, and the coordination and collaboration for the establishment of a functional global partnership among nations. These aforementioned goals are nothing short of overwhelming and staggering. They defy, they mock, they frustrate, they challenge, but, above all, they still provide an opportunity for the brotherhood of man to examine the existing inequities and blight of poor countries, and develop a strategic plan to improve the social and economic conditions of the world's most vulnerable and in need. This is both moral and right, if we truly hope to combat the pressing and depressing problems of the developing countries. Paradox has a face. And, the multiplicity of problems and challenges that the developing countries face will never improve without sacrifices by all involved – donors and recipients, national governments, technocrats, the people themselves – all must collaborate with commitment and will to create change. Without a sense of true togetherness and working and striving together, we would likely have to face a new declaration for needed reforms. That likelihood should be unthinkable!

Optimistic internationalism, therefore, must be the focus of the global response if there is any hope to improve economic growth and development towards sustainability, the triumph over diseases like HIV/AIDS, malaria, and tuberculosis, and the other complex diseases (the neglected tropical diseases) affecting the populations of developing countries.

The MDGs initiative is another start to trigger needed global reform and change, whether or not some of the goals are impossible to achieve within the anticipated timeframes, or ever, in some countries. I reiterate the absolute necessity for commitment and collaboration by everyone. Surely, we can expect the leaders and agents responsible for overseeing the MDGs to play a major role and influence the direction and progress of the program; but, they must not do so arbitrarily. The freedom given to the leadership to organize and prioritize must be limited by the needs of the populations to be served.

The MDGs, unfortunately, covered so many varied phases of progressive development for countries that were not realistically ready to embrace the goals that there was (or should have been) no surprise that many of the goals were not achieved in a manner to benefit many of the participating countries. That must not necessarily be considered either a negative or failure, but certainly contributes to frustration and disappointment to all involved with the daily operations. This stifles and kills enthusiasm commitment, and will.

The continuing dependency on donors remains extremely problematic, and had a distinct influence on many countries not coming close to achieving defined goals. This anticipation for funding based on a percentile formula of 0.7% of the gross national product (GNP) of donor countries for development assistance was hyper-optimistic. Granted, many donor countries made commitments in good faith and had the utmost intent to honor those financial disbursements to conform to the committed timeframes, but the evolving global economic distress and uncertainty put those hoped for funds into jeopardy. This clearly illustrates another disadvantage of planning longitudinally across a planet of over 6 billion people. It makes no difference whether or not the efforts or goals were a perfect vision of what is necessary to foster meaningful change, if the desired outcome is not accomplished. It reverts to just being an effort! While efforts can be applauded and celebrated, we need more than efforts and declarations. We need true and unified commitment and a renewed sense of togetherness, if we have any hope for "optimistic internationalism" to work and make life livable for the poor, hungry, and disadvantaged people of our globe.

Disappointingly, excerpts from a United Nations (UN) report indicate that: "At the midway point between their adoption in 2000 and the 2015 target date for achieving the Millennium Development Goals, sub-Saharan Africa is not on track to achieve any of the Goals. Although there have been major gains in several areas and the Goals remain achievable in most African nations, even the best governed countries on the continent have not been able to make sufficient progress in reducing extreme poverty in its many forms." The prevailing consensus is that, without a miracle, albeit, very unlikely, this trend will continue through 2015, and most likely beyond.

Conclusion

Regardless, whether one thinks or considers the MDGs, a sequel to Health for All 2000, or not, the MDGs, collectively, as a program, is without doubt, one of (if not), the most ambitious and ingenious approach, with defined goals and targets, ever undertaken to alleviate poverty, promote growth and development, seek health equity and control and prevent disease, advocate sustainability of the environment, establish solutions for child and maternal mortalities, and heighten global partnership for free and fair trade, while examining the needs of countries at risk and considerate options to correct inequalities.

Nonetheless, as we seriously assess the progress and likely outcome of the goals, a discouraging picture emerges. HIV/AIDS keeps on "galloping," defying comprehensive and asserted efforts to suppress and marginalize the disease. Malaria still kills someone in Africa every 30 seconds, and 1 in 5 childhood deaths in Africa are due to the disease. Insecticidal nets for beds are comparatively cheap and a great preventive measure against malaria, yet progress is slow in the distribution to have a serious impact on the continuing transmission of this disease. Tuberculosis remains a major disease of poverty, and continues as a problematic affront to public health globally, with about 1.8 million deaths annually. According to WHO, new infections occur at the rate of one per second worldwide, and while an infection does not often manifest clinically, the fact illustrates the widespread distribution of the tubercle bacillus, the causative agent, particularly so in countries challenged by maintaining a sanitary and hygienic environment, and the availability of resources for diagnosis, treatment, and prevention and control. The added factor of drug-resistant strains of the TB organism and the concomitant complications of clinical tuberculosis and AIDS infection, contribute to a depressing vista of the future.

Wars, famine, hunger, genocide, and a sense of hopelessness remain unabated in a world of continuous turmoil, unrest, and uncertainty. The attribution of environmental sustainability, national development, and the alleviation of poverty continue to be elusive and challenge our collective commitment and will, defying and mocking our ingenuity, at times. Mothers and babies still dying at increased rates in poor countries. Free and fair trade is really not fair or free, and trying to bring countries together to rectify the inequities is a big hurdle, despite the nicety of words and encouraging forecasts that emanate from international meetings. Many children still have no real access to primary or secondary education, and, if they do, it is mostly inadequate and provides little preparation for life's challenges, or vistas for opportunities to succeed in the job market. The global situation is depressing, but, never truly hopeless in a world of plenty, leaving one to ponder and wonder, where are we going from here? And, will hope ever truly shine by putting an end to inequalities! The stuttering comments coming from UN officials on the MDGs progress are insightful, evasive, and somewhat apologetic. And, while we have total empathy for goals that are intent to do good, another failed initiative is unacceptable. There is obvious fear that the outcomes hoped for would not be realized. The principles of the MDGs, however, whether or not reservations of their inflation were fair, established a template to work with and a track to follow to help the poor and dispossessed of the world look to better tomorrows.

Now that we are in the countdown phase of the MDGs to 2015, a reasoned question is, when will inequity end, and do we have the resources to end it? Do nothing. Let each country plan their destiny. We are not our brothers' keepers. Why should I care about the plight and blight of developing countries? They are all corrupt. They cannot manage or govern. None of the aforementioned applies to today's world. We are all in this together. Criticism, blind or objective, is not going to help now. The options do not allow broad alternatives, other than unity of purpose and goals for the future in an imperfect world. If we lived in an ideal world, we would have no need to discuss and objectify programs like the millennium development goals. Providing aid and assistance should not be viewed as noble or charitable, but as something that is in every human's best interest to make the globe a better place for all. In the 21st century, we certainly have the resources to plan sensibly to truly meet the needs of the developing countries, and, even though we have come to a fork in the road, should not mean we have to panic, and stutter our responses. We must re-assemble, and re-assess; failure to do is an injustice to so many who need our guidance and involvement to achieve the goals that can become a reality.

On the other hand, we must be admonished that we cannot continue along the path of spending years and resources to develop noble and needed goals, if they cannot be fulfilled. I referenced a return to the table is necessary – re-assemble – and consider reverting to the fundamentals of public health practice – safe water, food security, sanitation and hygiene, introduction of basic health care, prevention and control of the diseases like HIV/AIDS, malaria, and tuberculosis that paralyze so many in the developing countries, nutritional programs to conquer the indignity of malnutrition and hunger, massive vaccination programs to conquer preventable diseases, good governance to manager scare resources, commitment, and active collaboration with the people to be served, with the spirit that we are all in this as a unified force. There is no time for you and me – the theme is we.

A closing thought is that the current state of the world begs for the consideration of new ideas and true togetherness because the well-being of humanity is truly everybody's business. A debate as to whether that philosophical perspective is really applicable to the MDGs is senseless. A logical proposal is the regionalization of problems to improve functionality and maximize/optimize benefits. A case in point is sub-Saharan Africa as a model to work with, in spite of the differences of the many countries of the continent. This is a unique approach to respond to the region that has historically been identified with the major corrective needs, comparatively. Fortunately, there are many countries in Africa that are showing signs of measurable progress and success through commitment and sacrifice. We can begin with the countries that have been known to be most at risk and in need. That would be one category within the subset of a regionalization objective, and then follow with the same philosophy to ultimately include the entire continent. The same can apply to Asia, Latin America, and other sectors of the globe whose leadership is anxious to examine and apply new ideas and options to improve the lives of their people. In essence, the system entails a program of strategic, well-planned reasonable objectives that can be realized through collective collaboration and prioritization. This system, if adopted, would be less cumbersome, can be better managed, and with limited goals to achieve the most pressing needs of participating countries can be potentially more successful. One small step at a time is not unreasonable, regardless of whether the world that we live in is a plethora of serious problems.

I was just thinking playfully, using four words beginning with c – communication, collaboration, commitment, and consensus, contextual to the MDGs, and I want to amplify all four of these powerful words to make a point – sit at a posh pub in Nairobi, Kenya, a coffee shop in Lagos, Nigeria or San Jose, Costa Rica, a restaurant in Lahore, Pakistan, a family party in Caracas, Venezuela, a lecture at a university in Cairo, Egypt, or a roadside bar outside of Kingston, Jamaica, – ask those assembled in these diverse and different settings, with different cultures, traditions, hopes and aspirations about tomorrow, what do you think of the Millennium Development Goals? What percentage of those asked, what ought to be a very applicable and relevant question for their future well-being, will have any knowledge of the subject? Equally important and of logical consideration, is how many will associate a significant change in their lives, for the better, linked to an outcome of the goals? Successful initiatives demand true collaboration and buy-in. People must know what is being planned and instituted for their future. They have to be a part of it. They must, no pun intended, feel it!

My final and parting reflection of the MDGs is true ambivalence. I compliment and applaud those who gave us 8 goals that covered major elements of the global society and governance with the intent for reform and commitment for an improved quality of life and living, particularly for the most disadvantaged people on the planet, living in resource-poor countries, excessively vulnerable and at risk for most threats – education, economic development, health, environmental sustainability and social security. I also scold at the same time and chastise the same people for their blind optimism, confidence and idealism, at times, overlooking realism and compelling evidence of what can and cannot be achieved in a world of problems, burdened by inequities, mocking our sense of purpose and zeal, and leaving us all wondering and doubting, what do we do after 2015?

Nonetheless, and with a little residual reasoned optimism, the thought and hope for a forward-looking agenda for social change and health equity still persists and, hopefully, could conform to Arnold Toynbee's idea of "an age in which human society dared to think of the health of the whole human race as a practical objective." Or, to Bono's pleas for the forgotten poor, "hunger, disease, the waste of lives that is extreme poverty is an affront to all of us….that we do not treat this as an emergency-------that's our crisis." Amen.

"My peers in the developing world, however, don't have it quite so easy. Each day my colleagues confront the world's major microbial killers; the causes of acute respiratory infections and diarrheal diseases, tuberculosis, malaria, measles, pertussis, hepatitis B and C infections, neonatal tetanus, AIDS, and dengue fever. But, critically, they do so without any of the resources that I consider essential for the diagnosis and treatment of such infections. The sheer volume of patients, the deteriorating facilities in which they are diagnosed and treated, and, more often than not. The limited resources available, all serve to prevent the heroic practitioners of the developing world from accomplishing what they would be able to in more ideal circumstances. Their daily frustrations are no doubt far greater than mine are. It is the paradox of our era that while they struggle, we are so privileged that we are frequently unaware that their struggle exists."
Steven M. Wolinsky, M.D., Professor of Medicine
Northwestern University Medical School
In: Laurie Garrett's Betrayal of Trust: The Collapse of Global Public Health

"I'm like everyone else – I see the world in terms of what I would like to see happen, not what actually does."
Paulo Coelho, The Alchemist

Chapter 4

Water, Sanitation/Hygiene and Health

Introduction/Historical Background

The quest for clean water is as old as civilization, and evidence indicates it could have started in prehistoric times. Historical records also suggest that people throughout the ages took varied measures to assure that they had clean water to drink. This affirmation has been validated in Sanskrit writings approximately 2000 B.C. of the procedures applied to treat "impure" water – boiling, filtration, or storage in copper vessels exposed to sunlight. Additionally, biblical references confirm the customs of Hebrews about clean drinking water in general, and the early Judaic laws of the use of water for washing and cleansing before partaking of meals as a routine hygienic practice. Hippocrates, acclaimed as the "father of medicine", in his early writings and observations, exemplified by his treatise, "Airs, Waters, and Places," noted the differences in water quality in his search for a healthful source of water, and the concurrent influence of water on health, distinguishing problems faced by inhabitants who drank water from marshy areas in different seasons, whether summer or winter, and the impact on health.

The ancients, particularly, Greeks and Romans, have been recognized and praised in the annals of engineering and public health for their early innovations to assure a safe water supply to their populations, using water treatment technologies to control both odor and taste, a remarkable feat for the period. To consider that millennia later, we are still using methods and fundamentals that they established amplify their ingenuity and capability in their handling of water. The Italians just about perfected a sand filtration that has been in place for centuries and adapted for use throughout the developed world until the advent of the Industrial Revolution in the 19th century brought an entirely new set of perspectives and more sophisticated approaches to water treatment to conform to changing demands and needs of society.

This microscopic historical overview of water's societal role was intentionally brief, and only meant to amplify the most pertinent major evolutionary phases that took place over millennia to obtain and sustain a clean water supply globally. The objective of this short retrospective was to lead into the other broad and compelling aspects of clean water, which continues to be problematic in all countries, with few exceptions, but particularly to the resource-poor countries of the planet where close to one-fifth of the world's population continue to obtain their water from microbiologically unsafe sources at the advent of the 21st century. In the process, this factor contributes to threats to public health as waterborne diseases, with excessive morbidity and high mortality in some countries, exemplified by cholera and typhoid in environmentally degraded poor communities.

Water as a Global Resource

Freshwater is the planet's greatest natural resource that helps to ensure the survival of humanity and the sustainability of health. Interestingly, examining the totality of water as a resource, some surprising facts emerge. For example, only about 2.53% of the earth's water is fresh, the rest is seawater. In the last three decades, the reasoned consensus supported by environmental statistics and assessments and concurrent underlying concerns is that the earth's freshwater capacity is being threatened by population growth, misuse, and ecological degradation, and the growing alarms worldwide that if these trends continue many countries will face threatening water shortages as early as the year 2025. While this estimate might seem unduly overblown and pessimistic, the reality is that a water crisis has already been existence for decades, and will likely continue to be more problematic for most developing countries, accompanied by the concurrent severe consequences to society and health.

A study of the globe's population of 2.5 billion people in 1950, compared to the current global population of 6.5 billion, plus the predictions that by the year 2050, the human population is expected to be around 9 billion people, have become a cause for serious alarm and corrective action, pertaining to water and its usage. Obviously, the population growth in some countries defies intervention or easy answers, but the water quantity and quality problems can be marginalized and improved by managed priorities and commitment of national, international organizations like WHO and the World Bank, and NGOs. While the general impetus today continues to be aspects of water quantity, there is little doubt that water quality will become the central focus of the future because of the ubiquitous problems of water contamination as a hazard to public health, particularly in resource-poor countries. The quality impetus, however, does not rule the agenda fully, because quantity is of acute concern in many countries throughout the globe, exemplified by the rapidly growing economies of China and India, populated by about

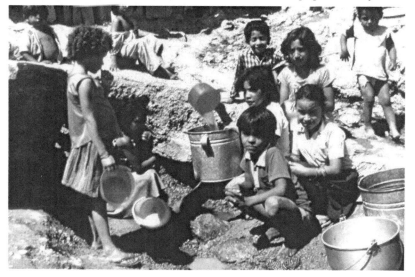

35 percent of the people of the world.

As indicated previously, a periscope of the world of over 6 billion people and about 200 countries as a unit or denominator is always reason for concern, because so often the numbers projected become suspect, not by intent to deceive, but by the mere circumstances of the difficulty in obtaining reliable data from many sources in developing countries. Often, much of the data accumulated from surveys, studies, and assessments are nothing but well-meant estimates. Since we live in a world of numbers, we continue to indulge by necessity in what is provided, and, I reiterate, as estimates only. The global health authorities indicate that over a billion people in poor countries have limited access to water, and nearly 3 billion have any access to essential sanitary facilities, conducive to health maintenance and promotion. While the minimum threshold for water averages about 20 liters, most people in developing countries access are limited to about 5 liters daily. Additionally, more than 700 million people (a conservative estimate) in 43 countries do not meet the water-stress threshold of 1,700 meters per person. Distressingly, and in spite of the many clean water prioritizing initiatives, this number is expected to be about 3 billion in 2025, and predominant challenges will be in the rapid expanding economies of countries like India and China, and just about all of sub-Saharan Africa.

In fact, clean water is a basic, if not the most basic human requirement. It is also specifically addressed in the MDGs to reduce by half the proportion of people unable to reach or afford safe drinking water. The challenge is titanic because more than a third of the world's population in the poorest countries has any access to safe water. In some countries, potable water constitutes 10 percent or less of the water supply. Unfortunately, like so many other aspects of assessing and making rationale determinants of MDG data from developing countries, water is no exception. Analyses from many developing countries illustrate the unreliability of data, even something as rudimentary as defining what "access" to safe drinking water means. Additionally, surveys that include information on access or availability of clean water in many countries are incomplete, sketchy, not uniform, and unreliable, confounding and compounding the disparities within countries and across regions of contiguous countries or continents. To amplify the problem, there is no one standard or defined criteria or methodology for determining water quality, and, surprisingly, even the definition of a safe water supply and sanitation differs from country to country. This creates another discount and barrier when attempts to achieve goals globally are evaluated for conformance to any established criterion or standard. The correction of so many basic deficits, therefore, is an absolute mandate, if we have the slightest hope of making a meaningful impact on the myriad problems linked to safe water, sanitation/hygiene and health.

In the future, both developed and developing countries that are committed to sustainability programs for clean water must consider a new water accounting framework as a policy option. The water footprint (the total amount of water used to produce goods and services consumed within a country) has emerged as a logical option. This would be a distinct improvement and more accurate measure than the traditional data on water use that countries have used, which heightens the concept of supply and usage by activity e.g. agriculture, industry, and domestic. The advantage of the water footprint indicator covers both demand and consumer use and is a more reliable measure that can be applied to determine the variables between countries and further establish guidelines to be achieved by nations, as countries accelerate their efforts to improve their water supply in a sustainable manner.

Water, therefore, is an absolute necessity that supports and enriches life and living. It is impossible to imagine living without water, especially clean water that is a major component of health, and environmental sustainability. Historical records indicate that the success of early settlements throughout the world was totally linked to the location and availability of water, and the disappearance and death of communities was associated with a decline or cessation of the supply of water. Man, in his wisdom, therefore, has historically established and set up habitation near water to ensure and support productive activities and subsistence. But, the regions of the world that are mainly challenged for providing an adequate and safe water supply for their inhabitants are most of the countries of Africa and Asia, burdened by burgeoning populations with outdated facilities/reservoirs, obsolete technology, and an infrastructure that is simply incapable of meeting the current and future needs of the people. Not surprising for the many public health advocates with an interest in development in Africa is the saying in many African countries that "water is life."

Water, Sanitation, and Hygiene:
Impact on Disease Transmission

For decades, it has been customary for public health journals and practitioners throughout the world to address sanitation and hygiene, either as entities, or quite often jointly in discussing the relevance to health and disease prevention and control. The annals of public health affirm this custom. Nonetheless, there are still many well-respected public health advocates who think that the separation is needed because sanitation (and hygiene in like manner) fails to receive the attention it deserves compared to water, and this deficit limits the potential for sanitary initiatives to have meaningful and measurable impact. Recently, however, the public health literature is treading new ground, and for good reason, to conform to a new progressive and more holistic movement by incorporating water to precede sanitation and hygiene, and in the process the introduction of a new acronym to the public health literature, WASH, highlighting the relevance of water (WA) to sanitation (S), and hygiene (H). It is not only truly innovative, forward-looking and logical, but serves to remind all of the important relationship and pertinence of water, not only as a composition of three-quarters of the earth's surface and elemental to life and existence in general, but to the other sub-sets of activities like its role in sanitation and hygiene, and ultimate relatedness to health maintenance and disease control and prevention.

The water supply of countries, sanitation and hygiene, are all intricately interrelated and are now and will continue to be addressed as a global health priority with the current and proposed efforts to institute uniform guidelines to meet global goals for clean water and improved sanitation and hygiene. Clarification and refinement of the use of sanitation and hygiene is necessary to preclude any chance of overlapping that will suggest synonymy. Sanitation has been historically defined from various perspectives to include and heighten the environmental, hygiene, and other overall relatedness to health. In this text, it will be amplified with specificity, but not totally, to denote dealing with the public health aspects of human waste with inference to the environment and disease causation. Hygiene will be used contextual to the preservation of health and disease prevention. Realistically, however, while these differences exist and must be highlighted, it is impossible to think of water, sanitation or hygiene without a definitive relationship to health. An inadequate supply of clean water, lack of sanitation facilities, and poor hygiene continue to be serious threats to morbidity and mortality in the poor countries of the planet. Disappointingly, the illnesses and deaths linked to water, sanitation, and hygiene (WASH) are all preventable with basic public health interventions, but still remain a constant affront to all developing countries, particularly the least developed of these countries, burdened by the concurrent challenges of environmental degradation, and infrastructural deficits.

Diarrhea

Global health estimates indicate that there are approximately 4.4 billion cases of diarrhea annually, causing about 2.2 million deaths, of which nearly 1.7 million are children under the age of five, contributing to a staggering and deplorable 15 percent of all children in this age category, predominantly in developing countries. Equally relevant and policy implicating for disease control public health initiatives is, as a disease entity, diarrheal diseases contribute to 4.3 percent of the total global burden of disease. That fact remains a compelling and challenging statistic for health officials in poor countries. Interestingly, epidemiological assessments have associated 88 percent of this disease burden to lack of clean water, poor sanitation, and inadequate hygiene, all mitigated and prevented by good governance, commitment and will, strategic planning, objective prioritizing, a functional public health infrastructure, and community involvement and togetherness.

It is not the intent of this discussion to delve into the specifics of diarrheal diseases that are of special concern to global health, like cholera, typhoid, shigellosis, or rotavirus that infect nearly all children living in tropical regions before the age of 2 years old. These will be discussed separately in other sections of the text. The current overview is generic and only meant to highlight the broad spectrum of the global health epidemiology linked to diarrhea associated with water, sanitation, and hygiene.

Intestinal Helminths and Schistosome Infections

Helminth (parasitic) infections transmitted through soil and other environmental sources linked to poor sanitation constitute some of the most defying afflictions of inhabitants in all developing countries. One report suggested that about 10 percent of the developing world's population is infected. That, without doubt, in consideration of the number of helminth/parasitic species involved, the varied avenues for potential transmission, and the large numbers of people constantly at risk of infection, does not in any way reflect true prevalence. A WHO estimate magnifies the reality of the ubiquity of the problem in one of their annual reports by stating that more than half of the world's population, or over 3 billion people are infected by "worms," and that at any given time, nearly 450 million are ill because of the association, mostly children. A research report by de Silva et al. on the global prevalence and distribution of helminth infections and schistosomes in 2003 validates WHO assessments with an impressive numerical overview: over 1 billion people are infected by roundworms (Ascaris lumbricoides), 795 million by whipworms (Trichuris trichuria) and 740 by hookworms (Necator americanus and Ancylostoma duodenale). The major areas of the geographic distribution of infections were sub-Saharan Africa and Asia, predominantly the world's two most populated countries, China and India.

The majority or nearly all schistosome infections (schistosomiasis), also known as bilharziasis or snail fever, affecting more than 200 million people in more than 75 different countries, are caused by the five major species (Schistosoma haematobium, S. intercalatum, S. japonicum, S. mansoni, and S. mekongi, and occur predominantly in sub-Saharan Africa, with lesser prevalence in parts of Asia and the Americas. Transmission of the disease occurs when people become exposed to water during washing, swimming, or collection from a source infested with the intermediate snail host. Cercariae from the infested schistosome are released from the snail and penetrate human skin, further entering blood vessels, passing through the lungs and then to the liver where the cercariae mature to adults.

Eggs of the infected schistosome are passed through urine or feces of infected people to the environment contaminating water sources and perpetuating the cycle of infection. Basic sanitation by people not urinating and defecating in areas close to water sources can be a major preventive measure. Humans become infected when their skin comes in contact with water that was initially contaminated with Schistosoma eggs. Additionally, education of people at risk to the elementary aspects of schistosomiasis transmission in endemic countries, for example, the hazard of man-made reservoirs, ponds, streams, rivers and lakes, and the presence of snails in these sources of water to the occurrence of the disease are vital to control.

Schistosomiasis is at the epicenter of tropical diseases, second only to malaria in socio-economic importance, affecting millions of people in the developing world, predominantly Africans and Asians, and leaving about 600 million people in the cycle of risk at the dawn of the 21st century. This disease amplifies the linkage of poverty and public health needs of developing countries where people use the same water source to drink, swim, bathe, urinate, and defecate. Especially distressing, if not depressing, is the thought that environmental conditions under which the disease continues to be endemic offer little hope that these practices would not persist.

Dracunculiasis (Dracontiasis, Guinea Worm Disease)

Dracunculiasis, is seldom used as a descriptive term outside of professional circles. The disease when referenced is commonly referred to as guinea worm disease, and in parts of Africa – the "fiery serpent." It is an incapacitating, painful, and preventable disease caused by a nematode parasite, Dracunculus medinensis, and is transmitted by drinking water that contains cyclopoid copepods (fresh water microcrustaceans) that carry the infective larvae.

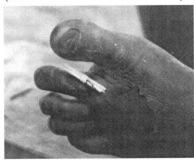

The disease is spread by adult female Dracunculus worms that emerge from the skin of the infected who enter sources of drinking water resulting in the release of infective larvae into the water. The larvae are then ingested by freshwater copepods (water fleas) that develop into an infective stage in about 10-14 days. People who are infected during this 10-14 day incubation period do not ordinarily manifest symptoms until approximately one year after the initial ingestion of larvae in contaminated water. At this stage of the infection cycle, a blister starts to form, predominantly on areas of the legs and feet, accompanied by itching, fever, swelling, and burning with intense pain at the site where the worm emerges. Ironically, many infected people in seeking relief of the itching and pain, immerse the infected part (mostly legs) in water like ponds and wells, permitting the female worm to release thousands of infective larvae and perpetuating the life cycle.

Prevention involves a safe supply of drinking water or something as elementary as filtering the drinking water through a cloth to remove the fresh water crustaceans. Concerted efforts by the Carter Center through the Global 2000 program, and collaborating organizations like WHO, UNICEF and CDC, "guinea worm" has been marginalized close to elimination, and, one day, hopefully eradication.

This disease was highlighted for a mixture of reasons and to illustrate that well-coordinated global public health initiatives can be successful with commitment, funding, and leadership. The disease has been endemic in many countries of Africa for centuries, infecting millions annually as late as 1986, and now there is ample reason for optimism the past and ongoing efforts could progress to eradication. It should also be of universal interest to note that "dracunculiasis is the only disease that can be eliminated completely by the provision of safe drinking water."

Trachoma

Trachoma is an infectious chronic inflammatory disease of the eyes due to a bacterium, Chlamydia trachomatis, causing swelling and redness of the eyes with discharges, scarring of the cornea, turning in of the eyelashes (entropion), corneal opacity, and conjunctivitis as the major clinical manifestation. Transmission is mainly from child to child in a school or home environment, or child to mother as applicable by the movement of disease spreading flies between individuals and by direct contact with infected eye secretions through "dirty" fingers and articles like towels, washcloths, and handkerchiefs. WHO reports that about half a billion people worldwide are at risk for the disease and 146 million threatened by blindness, and 6 million visually impaired by one or more of the changes following an initial infection – e.g. swelling of the eyelids, conjunctivitis, scarring due to corneal irritation etc

Trachoma is a perfect example of three concurrent interrelated deficiencies involving water, sanitation, and hygiene – lack of water, poor community sanitation (the presence of flies due to the lack of an effective control program), and lack of personal hygiene, due to a scarcity of water, to complete the transmission cycle. Trachoma has a link to poverty stricken countries where water continues to be close to a luxury, sanitation is poor, and hygiene lacking for many who are at risk for the disease.

Malaria

Malaria has been described in the annals of medicine more than 3,000 years ago, and remains a life-threatening and defiant disease today, with about half of the world's population still at risk of infection. While the disease is currently considered limited to the tropical belt of the globe, it should be of interest to recognize that at one time about two-thirds of the world's population were at risk. The disease is exclusively transmitted through the bite of an infected female mosquito of the genus Anopheles. It remains endemic in about 91 countries, or about half of the world's countries, and a continuous affront to global public health because of incapacitating morbidity and high mortality (close to about 400 million cases and over 1 million deaths annually), mostly on the African continent where 85 percent of all malaria deaths occur, and a child dies of the disease every 45 seconds, accounting for 20 percent of all childhood deaths throughout the world of which 90 percent are under the age of 5 years old. Countries of Asia and Latin America are also cause for rigorous prevention and control programs because inhabitants of these regions remain at risk due to an ecosystem that assists and perpetuates the vector's life cycle.

The disease is caused by species of the genus Plasmodium, of which Plasmodium falciparum and P. vivax are the most common of the four causative agents of human malaria. P. falciparum is the most problematic, because of the severity of illness in young children, non-immune adults, and tendency for higher mortality and complications linked to this parasite. The production of an effective vaccine continues to be elusive even in the midst of interim encouraging optimism of likely breakthroughs that could one day see a vaccine on the market. Control efforts and treatment are stymied by a growing drug resistance of anti-malarial medicine. The global public health community is forced to continue the traditional initiatives of reducing transmission by control of mosquito breeding sites and the elimination of varied sources of stagnant water, trash, and other forms of debris, including the approved use of larvicides, and the use of insecticide-treated mosquito nets, especially the efficacious long lasting insecticide impregnated nets, particularly in areas of potential high transmission.

The fidelity of public health in developing countries is again tested by the continuing inability of global health efforts to truly marginalize malaria. The disease has actually become a greater risk factor today than it was 30 years ago, creating a pressing economic burden in high incidence countries, affecting mostly the poorest of the poor, who can least afford treatment, and a true vista of the perils of poverty to the cycle of disease transmission and perpetuation.

Japanese Encephalitis

Japanese encephalitis (JE) is a disease caused by a flavivirus affecting animals and humans, and transmitted by mosquitoes belonging to the Culex groups, limited to countries of Asia, and the leading cause of viral encephalitis in Asia. The main hosts of the virus are birds like herons and egrets, from which the infection is passed on to pigs (by mosquitoes) where the virus amplifies in the newly infected pigs before transmission to humans that serve as dead-end hosts, contributing to an interesting arbo-viral zoonosis. The disease has an association with water and irrigation and extensive expansion of rice production during the crop planting and harvesting seasons. This becomes an ideal niche for the perpetuation of mosquitoes as the fields flood, and water becomes puddles. The control of the disease, therefore, involves the management of water resources used for irrigation, mainly in rice production, and the mosquito vector.

Most humans affected by the virus show no or only mild symptoms, but occasional cases, less than 1 percent of the total could be severely infected, and approximately 20 percent succumb to the disease, mainly young children without immunity. The disease continues to be reported from this region of the world, and during this writing (July 2010), cases that were highly suspicious of JE, were being investigated in India.

Hepatitis A

Hepatitis A (HAV), formerly called infectious hepatitis, is worldwide in distribution, and is an acute infectious disease of the liver, infecting about 10 million people worldwide annually. In countries of Asia and Africa, more than 90 percent of children by the age of six years may be infected, the majority showing no signs of the disease. The disease is highly contagious, spread almost exclusively by the fecal-oral route due to the ingestion of contaminated food and water. Like the majority of diseases in resource-poor countries, hepatitis A would likely be unreported. The estimated number of clinical cases annually is about 1.5 according to WHO (a conservative estimate in consideration of the population at risk). Young children under two years of age show no signs of infection, but adults over 18 years could manifest with icterus (jaundice), with concurrent nausea, dark urine, and light stools.

Hepatitis A can be prevented by vaccination, good sanitation and hygiene.

Arsenic

Arsenic contamination of groundwater has been found in many countries in disparate regions of the world, including the United

States. A reasoned assumption is that it is a far greater global health threat than previously envisioned, and worthy of epidemiological risk assessments of water quality, particularly in developing countries, because of the association of arsenic to various forms of cancer and serious skin conditions.

In the United States, the Natural Resources Defense Council (NRDC) evaluated data of the Environmental Protection Agency (EPA) in 2000, and determined that based on a study of 25 States, close to 56 million people were consuming water that contained unsafe arsenic levels that could contribute to a potential cause of disease. This analysis was presumably a sequel to a National Academy of Sciences (NAS) report in 1999 linking arsenic in drinking water to cancers of the bladder, lung and skin, and damage to the nervous system, heart, blood vessels, and skin problems.

Arsenic, however, became a serious concern to the world's public health community following the findings of natural contamination of Bangladesh's groundwater with high arsenic levels, exceeding 50 micrograms per liter, putting potentially more than 30 million people at risk (more than 20 percent of the country's population), and causing varying degrees of skin lesions, characterized by hyperkeratosis and melanosis, of about 1.5 million people. (It should be noted that WHO guideline level for arsenic is 10 micrograms per liter).

The arsenic contamination in Bangladesh is a study in irony. Tube wells were introduced about 30 years earlier as a safe system to preclude and minimize microbial contamination of the country's water supply that was considered to be a contributing source to the high prevalence of diarrheal diseases.

Fluorosis

The fluoridation of drinking water in the reduction of dental caries (decay) is considered one of the historical successes of health promotion and a credit to dental public health. While the proper supplementation of fluoride in drinking water has gained the recognition that it deserves, dental fluorosis, however, could develop in humans due to excessive prolonged ingestion of fluorine or its compounds, causing a white or brown mottled appearance of the enamel of developing teeth. Children in the age range of 1-4 years old are particularly vulnerable during this phase of tooth development. Additionally, long-term ingestion can also lead to skeletal fluorosis.

Drinking water remains the most common supply of fluoride, but other sources like food, excessive use of toothpaste, and exposure to air from industrial waste could contribute to clinical fluorosis (dental or skeletal) in regions that contribute to risk, even though the prevalence globally is not well defined, and in need of further studies and research that will provide a more comprehensive insight of the problem, and its public health pertinence and control.

There have been well documented linkages of high levels of fluoride with concurrent dental and skeletal fluorosis from known fluoride belts of land that include countries of North Africa, the Middle East, and Asia, including China where there is a high comparative incidence of both dental and skeletal fluorosis associated with drinking water, and possibly the high consumption of tea as a co-factor.

Discussion

For centuries, the public health community throughout the world recognized the significance of the relationship between water, sanitation, and hygiene (WASH), and the distinct association to health. As a point of information, the history of academic public health is replete with evidence that the early study and establishment of public health institutions in industrialized and developed countries were founded central to the consideration of the varied aspects of the provision of clean water, including the control of raw sewage contamination from entering the public's water supply, the treatment and processing of water to ensure safety as integral to early disease prevention initiatives, the practice of public health engineering, the

Don A. Franco

safety of food, and general principles of sanitation and hygiene. Interestingly, many of the early public health academic institutions were known simply as schools of hygiene. This early awareness and reasoned preoccupation with the importance of water, sanitation, and hygiene as potential sources to disease causation had a direct link to John Snow, a dedicated, well-known, and respected London physician, who in 1849, became an icon of environmental epidemiology, by proposing, with compelling documented proof - that cholera was a contagious disease. Snow's proclamation was two decades before the medical profession's acceptance of the germ theory of disease. This, without doubt, constitutes a fascinating and revolutionary accomplishment for medicine and public health, while giving credence to the role of surveillance epidemiology in disease control and prevention and emerging public health policy that serves us well to this day.

Snow's findings and association of cholera to water were that victims drew their water from the Thames River that supplied the Broad Street pump, and the water was collected below the point where the original contamination took place from this pump source. The conclusive public health message in Snow's work, still applicable to all countries, was the importance of a preventive system to modify the living conditions of the poor working class that would predispose them to contaminated water and the likely occurrence of cholera and other infectious disease outbreaks, linked to water and the environment. This, he theorized, can be achieved through enhanced sanitation and hygiene initiatives, particularly in poverty-stricken communities. The challenge continues in the 21st century where worldwide about 1 billion people (a conservative estimate) have no access to an improved water source (water supplied through a household connection, public standpipes, dug wells or protected springs), and an estimated 35 percent of the world's population, about 2.5 billion people, lack access to adequate sanitation and hygiene.

In most resource-limited countries today, the impressive accomplishments of Snow, over 160 years ago, is nothing but mythical or can barely be imagined. This is a form of irony that should mock and haunt us all in the 21st century. The majority of these countries are still incapable of supplying safe water, and adequate sanitation and hygiene – the very basic needs of humanity – leaving populations at risk to an innumerable number of diseases linked to these deficiencies. These poor countries, sadly, continue to commit the same offenses that Snow corrected 16 decades ago. It must be conceded that in the last two to three decades, more people in developing countries have had better access to safe water, sanitation, and hygiene; unfortunately, the progress and benefits of accessibility are negated by population growth, and, in the case of water, greater demand for use in the emerging agricultural and industrial sectors.

The problem of clean water remains and will likely remain extremely acute, but the global impact continues to amplify in the less advanced countries, through the paucity of sanitation by the lack of latrines, and the concomitant poor hygiene associated with limited or no hand washing facilities in many communities. These combined co-factors – scarcity of latrines and marginal or no hand washing access, including the use of soap, contribute to spread of infectious diseases, particularly linked to microbes transmitted through the fecal-oral route, as a result of food preparation, causing diarrhea, with infants and children at high risk. The concurrent potential morbidity and mortality outcomes associated with these varying forms of fecal exposure continue to be challenging to the poor countries of the globe, and a corrective action in need of greater immediacy.

The fact that 40 percent of people worldwide have no access to toilets and adequate sanitation and hygiene is or should be unthinkable today, and a compelling affront to global public health, even though the global public health community is convinced that improvements in both sanitation and hygiene are obvious pre-requisites to minimizing and reducing the enormous disease burden of developing countries. Equally important is that decision-makers and the political leadership in developing countries were cognizant of the need to improve and develop systemic programs to generate change. Historically, other pressing challenges and financial limits precluded any hopes of progress, regardless whether or not sanitary and hygienic interventions were about the most logical and cost-beneficial options to pursue. There seems no priority or strong advocacy for these sub-sets of public health.

The association of water, environmental sanitation and hygiene to global public health clearly demonstrates the monstrous problem that exists in most developing countries and the glaring mandate for providing adequate preventive programs that will curtail the transmission of pathogens and toxins to susceptible populations. The developed world has recognized for centuries, the attribution of clean water, sanitation, and hygiene as major forces in disease prevention and control. They have traditionally established successful and sustainable programs to assure these services to their populations. Sadly, in the majority of developing countries, there remains limited overt demand, in general, for these fundamentals to public health. Compared to the other needs of most developing countries, many, obviously, very pressing, nonethcless, the immediacy for public health correctives like safe water, sanitation and hygiene continue to suffer the indifference of benign neglect, with all the concurrent negative consequences to societies populated by the predominantly poor.

There are, doubtless, many reasons why this malaise in public health management and governance persists in so many resource-poor countries. The wide disparity in cultural, infrastructural, lack of commitment and will, and socio-economic deficits contribute to the problem, even though most of the people living under these conditions readily recognize and understand the risks that filth, improper disposal of waste, including fecal matter that is partially treated or untreated, contribute to increased transmission of pathogens and disease through contaminated surface waters, drinking water, and food by direct or indirect contact and the proven cause of an unacceptable total global disease burden.

Dr. Zafar Adeel, Director, the United Nations University, Institute for Water, Environment and Health (INWEH) in a reasoned preface in a report on the subject of sanitation as a key to global health (2010), summarized the challenges and reiterated problems that have been known for decades: "Water-related disease is responsible for a significant proportion of the global burden of disease....provisioning of adequate sanitation has not managed to keep up with population growth and the aggregate number of un-served people has increased.....sanitation is a critical component in striving for global equity and poverty reduction...disease transmission pathways demand that sanitation, hygiene and drinking water must all be dealt with to have impacts upon water-related diseases.....education, empowerment and community participation are equally critical.....coupled with national government support and programming.....There is a moral, civil, political and economic need to bring adequate sanitation to the global population – adequate for human health and adequate for ecosystem integrity."

Adeel's excerpts, examined from a current context, highlight, albeit realistically, the principles that have been presented at forums and symposiums worldwide for decades. While nothing truly novel has been offered in the quoted excerpts, the reiteration of what we already know is a good and necessary reminder. It serves to bite the conscience that so much still needs to be done. In fact, collectively, as a global public health community, we all seem to indefinitely repeat the niceties, benefits of public health promotion, and what we have to accomplish, but, we continue, unfortunately, to lose the race of change momentum to progress and success in many of the world's developing countries; many regressing instead of improving. And, the puzzling question remains, why!

Water, sanitation, and hygiene is more than disease-causing linkages to diarrheas, intestinal parasites and other "worms," trachoma, malaria, schistosomiasis, viral infections, arsenic contamination of water, fluorosis, and other acquired afflictions. They are vitally important, but nothing more than symptomatic of the broad and challenging spectra of public health inequities, particularly as they exist in the developing countries of the world. The initiatives and formally established goals for the provision of an adequate supply of clean water, sanitation, and hygiene throughout the planet, within a timeframe, entail both the maximization and optimization of a structured and integrated process across disciplines. This serves as a mocking defiance of reality based on the historical record, in spite of the best of corrective intentions. The poor funding of programs linked to water, sanitation, and hygiene, including the low level of prioritization for basic public health systems by both donors and recipients perpetuates this continuing dilemma that leaves poor countries underserved. The sung mantra that sanitation is vital to health, contributes to social development, is a good economic investment, helps to sustain the environment, and is achievable is not truly factored in with the resources needed to support a successful sanitary movement in developing countries that could truly contribute to reform and institute change. The resulting action never matches the passionate rhetoric!

Millions of people worldwide still defecate outdoors. The options are limited. The public health literature suggests that this practice equates to about 1 in every 5 persons on earth. This is something that simply cannot be conceived by decision-makers in the industrialized and advanced societies as they attempt to examine programs for funding, unless they or their representatives are on the ground and around the people in the villages and towns, and making on-site assessments of living conditions at the community level. Excreta and human contact becomes a way of life for so many – contributing significantly to the transmission of pathogens, the burden of disease, and the role of the environment in the cycle of disease.

The complex challenges of the poor countries of the world are obviously more than water. It is about rodents that contribute to plagues, mosquitoes responsible for malaria, dengue fever, and other arthropod-borne diseases. It is about the ubiquitous presence of cockroaches, filth, flies, and lice. It is about trash/garbage, sewage, microbes, and parasitic ova. It is about standing and pooling of water and replicating vectors of diseases. It is about no latrines and toilet paper and toddlers without diapers. It is about the perpetuating cycles of roundworms, hookworms, and tapeworms putting children at constant risk. It is about dirty bed sheets, bed bugs, and no mosquito nets. It is about contaminated food due to poor environmental hygiene and lack of refrigeration. It is about poor housing and gender inequality. It is about reasons for living with dignity and social justice. It is also about the need for continuing long-term commitment and programs for correcting the existing barriers to health and well-being of the poor.

Conclusion

An examination of the broad spectrum and impact of water, sanitation and hygiene (WASH) on health and disease globally, with emphasis on developing countries, provides mixed evidence, mostly not encouraging. Many of the existing conditions today are still deficient and downright depressing in about all of the least developed countries at the turn of the 21st century. Nearly half of the people living in the developing world continue to suffer from one or more of the major diseases linked to contaminated water, and poor sanitation and hygiene, with the concurrent potential of high morbidity and mortality, especially among children, who are immune deficient and most at risk. WASH programs must be addressed from the perspective of global poverty and economic development and growth to promote equity and improve the standard of living in developing countries as a prioritized focus, and integral to community life and living. The integrated process, if there is going to be any hope for sustained success, must be community-driven, regardless of resource dependency, and become part of a new sanitary revolution within developing countries. This must take the form of a unified voice to promote advocacy for the basic necessities like water, sanitation and hygiene that are cost beneficial and resource possible. Education, empowerment, collaboration, communication and the commitment of resources from national

Don A. Franco

governments and non-governmental organizations (NGOs) would enhance and assure success. In fact, everyone has to contribute to this formula for change and reform, without which, the inequities that exist today throughout the developing world will continue unabated, perpetuating the cycle of morbidity, mortality, nothingness and hopelessness, something that we, as a global community, cannot afford.

Life is an opportunity, benefit from it,
Life is a beauty, admire it,
Life is a bliss, taste it,
Life is a dream, realize it,
Life is a challenge, meet it,
Life is a duty, complete it,
Life is a game, play it,
Life is costly, care for it,
Life is wealth, keep it,
Life is love, enjoy it,
Life is mystery, know it,
Life is a promise, fulfill it,
Life is sorrow, overcome it,
Life is a song, sing it,
Life is a struggle, accept it,
Life is a tragedy, confront it,
Life is an adventure, dare it,
Life is luck, make it,
Life is too precious, do not destroy it,
Life is life, fight for it!
Mother Teresa, 1910-1997

Chapter 5

Infectious Diseases

(A) History
Background/Introduction

Throughout the history of civilization there were empirical observations that infectious agents could be responsible for certain diseases. Greek philosophers could be credited for their early contributions to the knowledge of many of the early theories of disease causation. They examined and rejected the theory that diseases could be caused by evil spirits when that concept was widely promoted and accepted by early medicine men and the church at the time. Just as compelling, the Greeks felt that the customary practice of the period, using magical words to cast a spell on patients, as a form of treatment, had no influence on the outcome of disease. The early Greek "medical establishment" during this period also associated what they considered the four elements of nature – air, fire, water, and earth to the human body, proposing philosophical similarities of those elements to man's four humors – blood, phlegm, black bile and yellow bile. Hippocrates, the "father of medicine," and an influencing force during this revolutionary period, and the cohorts belonging to his "school" theorized and taught that disease was nothing but an organized process that could be rationally understood and treated.

Early Greek medical literature also made reference to the knowledge of physicians in associating symptoms to a prognosis or disease outcome, and the use of the humors as a clinical supplement in their practice. This phase of the early development and growth of clinical medicine and practice continued until the advent of the Renaissance period (from about 1400-1750) that witnessed the founding and establishment of universities with medical faculties in many European countries and the teaching of formal courses in anatomy, including the emerging information from anatomical research, enhanced findings in pathology, and the introduction of new surgical instruments to enhance surgery, plus the invention of the microscope to facilitate research – contributing to a steady progression in the overall profession of medicine, and, as a result, the emergence of new concepts of disease causation and contagion.

The period of the Enlightenment that started in earnest around the 18th century on principles heightened during the "Age of Reason" introduced concepts of "modern" science and the social order of the world, including the use of scientific knowledge to improve living conditions. The value of experimentation was central to the period, and included the use of the microscope, and the early evolution of the study of the nature of infectious diseases contributing to an amplification of new scientific theories and information, and debunking the idea of the "humoral" theory promoted by the Hippocratic school, including many of the other non-scientifically proven concepts of disease.

The nineteenth century was of great historical significance and progression of knowledge, highlighted by the importance of disease transmission, including the modes of spread, exemplified by puerperal fever that threatened maternal and infant mortality. This early linkage of infection to childbirth introduced the concepts of the benefits of "scientific" bacteriology, and aspects of investigative epidemiology that helped to fuel the advances of the sanitary movement, and, doubtless, the initial efforts and success of vaccination as a mode of disease prevention that started in Europe at the time.

The twentieth century clearly reflected the continuation of rapid progress in all facets of the medical profession that was taking place throughout the world. This was demonstrated by the involvement of governments in most developed countries for the support of the new field of research, especially of infectious diseases, and the pertinence to causes, diagnoses and treatments of disease. This new optimistic impetus facilitated the role of university-based medical research and included the major hospitals and their staff in varied facets of infectious disease investigations that ultimately resulted in the development and education of an early cadre of specialists – those associated with infectious diseases, the epicenter of concern and importance to the medical profession at the time. This escalation of infectious diseases contributed to many concurrent dramatic advances in bacteriology, parasitology, pathology, and clinical medicine, because of the association of these disciplines to disease causing agents. This development and progressivism also helped to move forward the potential for treating diseases successfully, and a sense of excitement that the advancement of medicine has no boundaries, and we are living in an age that answers through research are possible, heightening optimism for the future.

The fact that optimism and growth of knowledge was at the epicenter of infectious diseases at this time, the world of medicine (and infectious diseases), nonetheless, is fraught with irony. During the mid 1970s and prior to the characterization of the human immune deficiency virus (HIV) association with AIDS in the early 1980s, many in the medical world of the industrialized countries had started to think, albeit prematurely, that the era of infectious diseases as a significant concern or threat to populations was coming to an end. At least, this was considered rational for people in the developed countries. The eradication of smallpox, the miracle of antibiotic use contributed to that reasoned optimism. Many academic institutions were considering re-defining their priorities pertaining to infectious diseases to conform to the emerging trend. This was obviously premature. HIV/AIDS entered the stage in the early 1980s and created new challenging dimensions for disease control and prevention, and a lesson that infectious diseases lie beyond the realm of a periscope. Their nuances are far too complex to predict with any degree of certainty, leaving us today just as challenged as the early pioneers were in creating a controlling force to deal with the complicated and unknown threats of infectious diseases, including the problem of antibiotic resistance and the new emerging diseases that are intent to challenge and confront our collective ingenuity.

Don A. Franco

Highlights of Infectious Diseases – Major Contributors
1600-2010

Antony (Antonie) van Leeuwenhoek, born in Holland in 1632, developed a passionate interest in small life (animalcules) and microscopes, and had a great influence in the progress of biological discoveries by his careful and meticulous observations of different specimens, including the first descriptions of bacteria and protozoa, gaining the accolade, "the Father of Microbiology." His early research and quest for knowledge gave the world of science both the lives of things unseen by the naked eye ("little animals") and the benefits of the microscope to new discoveries and medicine.

Edward Jenner, born in England in 1749, related to nature from his boyhood, and developed an affinity to medicine, which he practiced after his graduation from medical school in a rural farming community, treating mostly farmers of the region, many who worked with cattle and other livestock. During the period that Jenner practiced, smallpox was rampant and a major cause of epidemic outbreaks and death. His keen sense of observation as a practicing clinician in a farming community was beneficial – he found that many of his patients who had worked on cattle farms and developed cowpox, a relatively mild disease, never developed smallpox, a disease of both high morbidity and mortality.

Jenner was anxious to confirm experimentally his clinical observations, and when a young milkmaid came to be treated with classical symptoms of cowpox (sores and blisters on hands), he extracted liquid from her sores, and liquid from a patient with a slight case of smallpox. Jenner was resorting to the "fundamentals" of disease transmission, control, and immunization for his answer. He wanted to inject someone with an extract from the cowpox liquid to determine and confirm whether it would protect the person from the more serious and "killer" disease, smallpox.

Jenner got a local farmer to agree with his theory of "inoculation" and poured the liquid from the cowpox infected person into the scarified arm of the farmer's son, who subsequently came down with cowpox in a mild form. The farmer's son recovered quickly, and six weeks later Jenner then used the same procedure and injected him with the smallpox liquid. To the relief of Jenner (and the family of the young man), the son showed no signs of smallpox, and the genesis of vaccination (from the Latin, vacca – cow) to the world of medicine and public health.

Ignaz Semmelweis (1818-1865), a Hungarian born physician, specializing in obstetrics, introduced the medical world to the concept of antiseptic prophylaxis in maternal care during childbirth, prior to the development of the germ theory of disease. Semmelweis showed that puerperal or childbirth fever, a cause of excess mortality of mothers at the time, could be drastically reduced by proper hand washing of care givers during obstetrical delivery. While his theory met initial resistance by many in medical practice in Vienna at the time, the results over time were impressive, leading to vindication and acceptance of the practice of proper hand washing. The death rate of women giving birth in maternity wards of hospitals fell from a high of 30% to 0.85% by the simple practice of this introduction of hygiene.

Semmelweis's theory, like many of the early successes of infectious disease epidemiology of the period, was based on nothing but mere observation. He found that doctors and medical students assigned to maternity wards that did not wash their hands after being in the autopsy room and subsequently treated patients, put pregnant women about to give birth to high risk of infection that contributed to excess mortality. His work has benefitted the control of infectious diseases as pioneering for centuries, yet, in the 21st Century, many maternity patients in developing countries still die needlessly from similar infections – ranging from the lack of clean water or water – period!, antiseptics, the use of surgical gloves, proper antibiotic therapy, and clinic/hospital acquired infections.

Louis Pasteur was born in Dole, France, in 1822, into the household of a poor family. Being comparatively poor, however, did not in any way deter his early quest for knowledge that allowed him to gain entrance and degrees from some of his country's most prestigious educational institutions. Later in his career, his devotion and academic acumen led to professorial appointments in chemistry and science at elite universities in France. His impressive research and experimentation in the diverse fields of chemistry and medicine highlighted his personality – patience, highly inquisitive, and the innate ability to correlate research data to hypotheses and linking the overall results to solve "real world "problems.

Pasteur debunked the accepted theory at the time that the emergent growth of bacteria in broths was not due to spontaneous generation, but to the presence and replication of micro-organisms that caused fermentation. The living organisms that caused the broths to change and ferment came from the outside, in the form of contaminants like dust containing bacteria and spores. Nothing will grow in the broths unless the flasks were open permitting the entrance of living organisms. This experiment not only put an end to the advocacy of spontaneous generation, but was the genesis of the germ theory of disease. The inference was clear – if "germs" can cause fermentation, they can cause infectious diseases.

The applicability of Pasteur's research findings has had influence on the global scene to this day. His experimental diversity and commitment to detail proved that micro-organisms contributed to the spoilage of milk, beer, and wine. His heat process treatment of milk to kill organisms that could ultimately ferment and spoil milk was responsible for the expansion of the early dairy industry in Europe. That effective heat process is known throughout the world as pasteurization in his honor.

As implied, Pasteur's research work and experiments were so diverse for the period that it approximated being unbelievable the amount that he actually accomplished. His passion and determination could be the result of having lost three of his five children to typhoid fever. He was, therefore, intent on obtaining answers to prevent diseases and death. He acquired a missionary zeal in the process, and worked with Joseph Lister (to be addressed next) to introduce antiseptic precautions to surgery to prevent micro-organisms from entering the bodies of surgical patients that could potentially cause complications leading to infection and death.

Pasteur's early work on immunity and the role of vaccines to prevent diseases included his extensive investigations into cholera in chickens, the production of a vaccine for anthrax in cattle, and the first vaccine developed for control of the deadly rabies virus, which was always fatal in humans, mostly associated with bites from dogs affected with the virus.

Pasteur died in 1895, near Paris, having left a legacy of contributions to the advancement of chemistry, medicine, and the art and science of vaccinology that has benefited the world in myriad ways to this day. The full extent of his impact and achievements on both society and medicine has been affirmed. Additionally, his accomplishments planted seeds for the continued progression that was taking place in medical research at the end of the nineteenth century. The world has been grateful, and his name immortalized for the lives saved and the diseases prevented by his committed professionalism to experimentation, research, and medicine.

Joseph Lister was born in England in 1827, and displayed an affinity for science from early in life that further led to a degree in medicine and surgery with outstanding academic accomplishments. Bleeding, pain, and infections were affronts to surgery in Lister's era. In Scotland at the Edinburgh hospital where Lister practiced with his father-in-law, a distinguished professor of surgery, nearly half of the surgical patients died from complications linked to infections. In many hospitals throughout Europe, the death rates associated with surgical infections exceeded that experienced in

Scotland. Lister was intent and fully dedicated to finding ways to minimize the "inevitability" of infection.

Lister recognized from observations that simple fractures healed readily; but, patients with compound fractures where the bone protrudes from the skin and become exposed to air had an excessive death rate. Concerned about the need to correct this disparity in surgical infections, Lister, while a professor of surgery at the University of Glasgow, read of Pasteur's work of "germs" from the air that could cause infection, and was convinced that if organisms entering the surgical wound could be prevented or killed, infection could be prevented. Lister then resorted to the use of a carbolic acid (phenol) solution to swab wounds, wash his hands and instruments, and apply to bandages after surgery. His accumulated data on the attributes of antiseptics, exemplified by carbolic acid, as a deterrent to surgical infections was so impressive that the findings were published in the iconic medical journal, the Lancet in 1867.

Many of the evolving new innovations in medicine at the time were not readily accepted, and Lister's introduction of antisepsis to surgery was no exception, and, as a result, acceptance was slow, because of that continual tendency of many physicians at the time to resist change. Lister, however, never

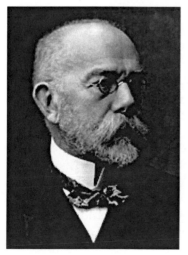

lost his composed confidence, nor was he discouraged by the indifference of some surgeons to his concepts. Over a period of time, nonetheless, Lister's theory of antiseptic surgery had gained acceptance throughout the industrialized world, accompanied by numerous academic honors and awards for his contributions to medicine and surgery. He died in 1912, but has left us with what remains today the most effective tool of surgery – the control of infection through antiseptic principles.

Robert Koch was born in Germany in 1843, and showed early academic brilliance from his childhood. He pursued studies in natural science and then medicine at the University of Gottingen, where he obtained his medical degree in 1866. During medical school, Koch had the good fortune to be exposed to dedicated researchers like Professor Henle, who published early work on contagion, and, doubtless had an influence on the direction that Koch took in the field of medicine.

Koch's major accomplishments and contributions to medicine followed the path of research in bacteriology. While he saw and treated patients, he was fascinated by laboratory work, and he used his microscope to great advantage to discover more about the diseases that plagued his patients. One of these diseases, anthrax, a disease of cattle and sheep, was widespread in Germany at the time, and was transmissible to humans, causing severe morbidity and mortality. Koch examined the blood of infected sheep with anthrax microscopically, performing scrupulous investigations in the process, and discovered that the disease was caused by a bacillus that formed spores. He also described the techniques used to isolate the organism, contributing to a growth and development period in the expansion of bacteriology in medicine and clinical practice.

Koch established the four basic fundamentals that become the cornerstone of modern bacteriology, known as Koch's postulates, heightening the concept of the germ theory of disease that affirms an organism to be pathogenic or disease-causing. The postulates are: (1) The bacteria must be found in every case of the disease; (2) The bacteria must be isolated from the host with the disease and grown in pure culture; (3) The cultured organism must be able to be transferred to a healthy susceptible host who will show signs of the disease; and (4) The organism must be recoverable from the experimentally infected host. Koch, therefore, became the first person to demonstrate that a specific organism was the cause of a disease. In the process of experimentation with bacteria, he also became the first researcher to grow bacteria in colonies, initially on potato slices, and later on Petri dishes with solid gelatin media.

Koch, at a scientific meeting in Berlin in 1882, announced that the cause of tuberculosis, a disease that was one of the major causes of death in Europe at the time, was due to a microbe and was infectious. Other scientists had implied that this was so without validation; still, others had reservations. But, Koch impressed his colleagues that his published findings met the criteria defined in his postulates, amplifying his role as both an outstanding research bacteriologist. As a physician, he was an early contributor to public health practice by promoting hygiene and legislation to control infectious diseases.

Koch's knowledge and fame became "transparent" to the world of diagnostic bacteriology and medicine, and he was invited to present his theories and assist disease control efforts in Egypt and India, two countries challenged by the deadly effects of cholera at that time. Although Pasteur had speculated that cholera was likely due to an organism, it was still to be validated. In Egypt, Koch did identify microscopically a comma-shaped organism from the stools of the infected, and these findings were later replicated in India, affirming the cause – effect of the microbe, Vibrio cholerae, to cholera.

Robert Koch's enthusiasm for finding answers through medical research could not be contained. This was exemplified by his discovery and description in 1882 of the organism that causes tuberculosis, including the infectious characteristics of the organism. This contribution to the "revolution" that was taking place in medical research at the time, specifically his work with tuberculosis, including efforts to prevent the disease, remains the historical icon in the world of medical microbiology, earning Koch the Nobel Prize in 1905 for his work.

Koch died in 1910 at the age of 67. Like all early researchers who contributed to the rapid advancements of medical science, Koch made mistakes and suffered his share of disappointments. His professionalism, nonetheless, established a path for public health medicine, research, and disease control and prevention for all to emulate.

Paul Ehrlich was born in Germany of Jewish ancestry in 1854. From an early age, he showed an affinity for science and medicine, with a unique interest in staining of microscopic slides in the university's medical laboratory. His devotion and work on staining was foundational for the emerging field of hematology and microscopy during that period, and included a method for staining, Mycobacterium tuberculosis, an acid-fast organism (not decolorized by an acidic rinse after staining), a diagnostic characteristic of the causal agent of tuberculosis, a leading cause of death throughout the world at the time. Ehrlich and co-researchers also did extensive work on infectious diseases that included a serum for diphtheria, a cause of high morbidity and mortality during that period and new innovations in chemotherapy by his discovery of a chemical compound, atoxyl, to treat sleeping sickness.

Ehrlich's legacy will be celebrated in medical history for his collaboration with his Japanese student, Sahachiro Hata, and the discovery of compound 606, Salvarsan (arsphenamine), in 1909, for the treatment of syphilis. Shortly after this chemical milestone, Salvarsan enjoyed widespread clinical use, and became the most widely prescribed drug in the world because of its effectiveness for treating syphilis and other infections, prior to the advent and availability of penicillin in the late 1940s commercially.

Ehrlich was a co-recipient of the Nobel Prize in Medicine in 1908 for his innovations and contributions to therapeutic medicine and research, and died of a stroke in 1915 at the age of 61.

Hans Christian Gram was born in Copenhagen, Denmark in 1853. He developed a keen interest early in life in subjects like botany and science that provided opportunities to work with the microscope and explore the unknown. His exposure to matters of science, doubtless, led to an interest in medicine, graduating in 1883. He travelled extensively throughout Europe and worked in the fields of pharmacology, bacteriology, and internal medicine.

Gram's accomplishments and contributions to medicine were in the emerging science of diagnostic microbiology studying blood and diseased tissues, and, specifically, methods for staining bacteria. He discovered that on microscopic examination of lung tissue from patients who died of pneumonia, for example, bacterial cells like pneumococci, associated as causal agents of the disease, had a distinct affinity for certain stains used for diagnostic purposes. Using Ehrlich's protocol of aniline water and gentian violet solution, followed by treatment with Lugol's solution (an iodine solution) and ethanol, Gram observed that some bacteria retained the stained color of the dye (Gram positive), while other did not (Gram negative). This method for distinguishing types of bacteria put Hans Christian Gram into the iconic world of microbiology and infectious diseases, establishing a standard procedure in use throughout the world today to distinguish two major classes of bacteria. He died in 1938.

Richard Julius Petri was born in Germany in 1852, and graduated in medicine in that country in 1875. Petri did his major work in bacteriology, and while working on tuberculosis, he wanted to improve on Koch's techniques for cultivating microorganisms. He invented what is known and used globally in microbiology and medicine, the Petri dish. The "dish" is made up of two flat double dishes of 10-11 cm in diameter and 1-1.5 cm high. The upper dish serves as a lid and prevents contamination from airborne microorganisms. The lower lid contains gelatin agar on which infectious material is inoculated and observed for growth, and subsequent observation of the bacterial colonies. This contribution by Petri helped to revolutionize bacteriology and introduced what is basically a simple device for the culture of microorganisms on solid media used in laboratories throughout the world today, with little or no modification of the original concept. The procedure has become a significant adjunct to bacteriology and an important supplement for the diagnosis of infectious diseases and public health practice. Petri died in 1921.

Dmitri Ivanovski was born in Russia in 1864. He enrolled at the prestigious University of St. Petersburg in natural sciences, developing a strong interest in diseases that affect tobacco plants, specifically, a new disease of tobacco plants destroying crops in the Crimean region of the country, called tobacco mosaic. He developed an experimental design to investigate the cause by crushing the infected leaves of tobacco into an "emulsion" that would pass through a bacterial filer, thereby, eliminating bacteria as a likely cause. The emulsified material that passed through the filer was, therefore, free of bacteria and was applied to the leaves of healthy tobacco plants by brushing. This process caused disease and the obvious deduction by Ivanovski that whatever caused the disease had to be either a toxin or an infectious agent smaller than bacteria.

Like a lot of early research as science continued to expand during this period, Ivanoviski's work did not get the recognition, regardless of the significance of his findings that an infectious agent other than bacteria, and proven smaller than bacteria, was proven to be involved, his results had no traction. He died in 1920, and it was left to a Dutch botanist, Martinus Beijerinck, to repeat his experiments that resulted in the genesis of a new life form to the world of microbiology, smaller than any organism previously described – the virus – the first to be recognized, and the cause of tobacco mosaic.

Martinus Beijerinck was born in Amsterdam (Holland) in 1851, devoting his professional career to teaching and research in agricultural and industrial microbiology, predominantly soil microbiology, and aspects of botany. He validated in 1898 the filtration experiments started by Ivanovski, affirming the linkage of a virus to tobacco mosaic disease, and subsequently gaining the accolade of the founder of virology for his accomplishments.

His extensive scholarship as researcher and teacher at the Laboratory of Microbiology at Delft which he founded, contributed to major discoveries varying from the process of nitrogen fixation that converted nitrogen gas to ammonia that can be used by plants, the role of sulfate-reducing bacteria, and the enrichment culture to study microbes from the environment.

While Beijernick did no known work in the study of disease and human virology, his research findings and validation that a virus causes disease in plants, exemplified by tobacco mosaic disease, and the evidence that viruses multiply in actively growing tissues and cannot replicate like bacteria, opened a new vista of knowledge that has a dramatic impact on the world of medicine forever. His introductory work set the stage for the new and exciting field of virology as a significant adjunct to infectious diseases in humans. He died in 1931.

Walter Reed was born in a small town in rural Virginia in 1851, the youngest of five children of a Methodist minister and his wife. His father's ministry brought him to Charlottesville, VA., there Walter had the opportunity to study at the University of Virginia, the institution founded by President Thomas Jefferson. At the university, he completed the academic requirements for the degree, Doctor of Medicine at age 18, a record that stands to this day as the youngest graduate in the history of the university's School of Medicine, and, likely, one of the youngest graduates ever in an American School of Medicine.

Reed continued his studies in New York City at Bellevue Medical College at the time and obtained a second degree in medicine from that college. He had no interest in the general practice of medicine, and pursued a career in the Army Medical Corps with different postings throughout the country, mainly in the west. Military medicine provided him the opportunity to further his studies at Johns Hopkins University in bacteriology and pathology, subjects of importance to the army disease control initiatives, and his overall medical responsibilities in the army. Reed also took advantage of joint faculty appointments that allowed him to research diseases, mostly infectious and exotic in nature, and networking with academic medical researchers in the Washington/Baltimore corridor, something that the military encouraged because of the obvious benefits of ongoing collaboration in disease prevention and control efforts.

In 1899, Reed traveled to Cuba to study typhoid disease, a serious health hazard to both the army and public at the time, and later became involved with the study of tropical diseases in general, and, with emphasis on yellow fever, a challenging cause of death in the region at the time. The existing thinking of the cause of yellow fever prior to Carlos Finlay, a Cuban doctor, was due to fomites through some form of human contact – clothing/bedding etc. Finlay, however, as early as 1881, proposed the theory that the disease was most likely transmitted by mosquitoes. This theory was both unique and revolutionary for the period, contradicting the traditional concepts of what were considered the ways how diseases were transmitted.

In the interim, the U.S. military losses in Cuba during the 1890s invasion were far greater for yellow fever than the deaths incurred in military activities. Walter Reed and his medical cohorts, charged to control these tropical and exotic killer diseases, examined Finlay's thinking and confirmed and validated the mosquito linkage, becoming the first to demonstrate that a mosquito could transmit a virus through biting of susceptible hosts to cause yellow fever.

This yellow fever causation concept of Finlay, heightened by Reed's collaboration and confirmation of the role of the mosquito, helped William Gorgas, a United States Army physician, and former U.S. Surgeon General, establish yellow fever control programs during the building of the Panama Canal, saving numerous lives in the process, and a definite adjunct to the completion of the "Canal."

The mosquito associated linkage to yellow fever brought new knowledge and insights to the study of infectious diseases that impact medicine throughout the globe today, and the role of vectors in general in disease transmission, especially in the tropical regions of the world. In retrospect, Finlay-Reed, thus, gave the world of medicine a new path to follow by their introduction of a hitherto unsuspected vector, the mosquito, as a serious hazard to health, particularly in the tropics to this day.

Unfortunately, Walter Reed, dedicated doctor of the United States' Army Medical Corps, died in 1902, following surgical complications of an appendectomy from peritonitis, but left a legacy for all in the world of infectious diseases and public health to celebrate – the saga of the mosquito's role as the cause of yellow fever.

(History has been overly kind to Reed's role in yellow fever's cause – effect and control, amplifying him in the discovery process. Dr. Reed's own publications have cited Dr. Finlay with credit for the discovery. As a result, I resort to joint recognition of both these contributors by using Finlay and Reed as examples of successful disease collaboration that benefits medicine and mankind).

Sir Alexander Fleming was born in Scotland in 1881. He enrolled at St. Mary's Medical School of London University, graduating with distinction in 1906. He served in World War 1 in the British Army Medical Corps, and at the end of the war returned to his Alma Mater (St. Mary's) to teach bacteriology to medical students. A part of his responsibility at the medical school was research. He conducted extensive studies on antibacterial substances, one of which was lysozyme, an enzyme which he found in saliva and other secretions, with antibacterial properties in 1922.

One day, during routine work in his laboratory in 1928, Fleming was working with Petri dishes, cultures, and infectious material, and was in the process of discarding some of the used Petri dishes with culture, and made an unexpected discovery – the presence of mold growing on a staphylococcus culture plate. The mold, surprisingly, appeared to kill the bacteria, a finding of compelling interest to an academic bacteriologist. Further experimentation proved the mold to be a fungus, Penicillium notatum, the precursor of the antibiotic penicillin, one of the ultimate discoveries of the 20th century that helped to change the course of medicine and chemotherapeutics.

Sir Alexander Fleming was knighted by the British Empire in 1944, and shared the Nobel Prize in Physiology or Medicine in 1945 with Ernst B. Chain and Howard W. Florey for their work with penicillin.

Walter Gilbert (1932-) and Frederick Sanger (1918-?) moved the world of genetics into another tier by their work with DNA sequencing to identify and determine the specific order of the nucleotide bases – adenine (A), guanine (G), cytosine (C) and thymine (T) in a molecule of DNA. The science of DNA is integral to the progress of basic biological research in the varied fields of medical diagnostics, forensic biology, biotechnology, and applied and basic research in general.

Gilbert of Harvard University, and his graduate student, Allan Maxam, and Sanger of England's University of Cambridge developed DNA sequencing methods in the early 1970s. This sequencing permitted the use of purified DNA directly, making it possible to read the nucleotide sequence for entire genes. New advanced technologies are now in vogue, but with the pioneering research contributions of these researchers in this challenging field, we can now move forward to look at the cell, the microscope, Mendel's work with genes/DNA, bacteria, viruses with a greater sense of appreciation. Inheritance, the genetic code and engineering that permits insight to the makeup of people, including the inheritance of diseases like cystic fibrosis, diabetes, mental retardation/Down syndrome, hemophilia, gene transfer of cells to cure or prevent diseases, the role of genes in cancer development or suppression, genetics in agriculture, fingerprinting for specific identification, biotechnology, and mapping the genome – with the potential for answers to the prevention and control of infectious disease - will all continue to progress because of the early search for answers by committed scientists.

The revolutionary contributions of Gilbert and Sanger to medical research and science brought with it recognition and prestigious awards to both – the Albert Lasker Medical Research Award in 1979, and the sharing of the Nobel Prize in chemistry in 1980.

Kary Banks Mullis was born in North Carolina in 1944. After showing academic brilliance and scientific inquisitiveness early in life, he went on to complete his PhD requirements in 1972. This was followed by faculty appointments at major academic research institutions and the challenges of the emerging field of genetics. He joined the Cetus Corporation in California in 1979, as a chemist, doing research on nucleotide synthesis. While at Cetus, Mullis in 1983, examined a method of finding and amplifying tiny fragments of DNA – the polymerase chain reaction (PCR) – a process that multiplies a single microscopic strand of the genetic material billions of times within hours. PCR basically permits the analysis of any short sequence of DNA or RNA that contain the minutest quantity of the molecules. The fact that the procedure can be done in test tubes, is highly efficient, and takes only a few hours, during which time unlimited numbers of copies of DNA (or RNA) can be made, heightens the valuable applicability of PCR. Mullis in a peer review article describes the PCR attributes best: "Beginning with a single molecule of the genetic material DNA, the PCR can generate 100 billion similar molecules in an afternoon. The reaction is easy to execute. It requires no more than a test tube, a few simple reagents, and a source of heat."

Mullis left Cetus in 1986 to join another research laboratory, and shortly after his departure the Cetus Corporation patented his PCR innovation in 1987. Mullis' initial work with PCR was a significant and important accomplishment and helped to open up the research windows into genetic mapping and the human genome. This exciting feat of Mullis has broad implications for various fields of genetics and medicine, making it easier to identify disease causing organisms that are difficult to culture, and, in the process, easier identification of bacteria and viruses, the diagnosis of genetic diseases, forensic investigations – medical or criminal in scope, and an essential tool for microbiologists throughout the world.

It should be of interest to note that Kary Banks Mullis, a well-respected research chemist/geneticist and recipient of the Nobel Prize in chemistry in 1993 for his work with PCR, was a man who did not fully accept or follow the traditional or accepted theories readily. He vigorously challenged the prevailing opinion of the world's medical community by refuting the causal association of HIV and AIDS. He also openly debated the accepted hypotheses of the social and natural scientists linking the destruction of the ozone layer to chlorofluorocarbons and gases from industrial waste and other environmental degradation factors to global warming. In essence, Mullis can never be considered anything but different, exciting, and provocative in scientific circles, because he only embraced theories that he considered complied with the principles and dictates of scientific proof, and was always prepared to heighten the subject with point – counter point to benefit scholarship, and, obviously, in his opinion the enhancement of knowledge.

Research with the human genome to advance science is inspirational and people involved tend to be passionate, focused, and downright competitive. Work with the human genome started in 1990 with the clear intent to gain insight and understand the genetic makeup of man, and the advantages that this acquired information will bring. This initiative was called the human genome project (HGP).

The first successful complete genomic sequence, however, was a map of the bacterium, Hemophilus influenzae, a free-living organism, using a method called whole genome shotgun sequencing that sequenced in less than a year the 1,749 genes of the bacterium and the concurrent assembly of unselected pieces of DNA from the whole chromosome that resulted in the complete nucleotide sequence – 1,830,137 base pair (the "rung" of a DNA double helix, made of one base from each strand, joined in the middle by a chemical bond.)

The success linked to this initiative depended on the cooperation and collaboration of researchers from academia, government, and the private sector, the latter exemplified by the Institute for Genomic Research (TIGR), located in Rockville, Maryland, that provided nearly half of the sequences. The reality of doing research of this nature, complex and expensive, was the acceptance that no one group could have done it alone. The findings of the H. influenzae sequence were first published in the scientific literature in 1995. It opened new vistas and became an impetus for global scientists involved with facets of genome mapping, including research with other organisms and the identification of complete genomes of many pathogens. This could contribute to new knowledge of diseases and assist in the manufacture of new vaccines for disease control and prevention.

The successful mapping of H. influenzae, doubtless, energized the vision of scientists working with the human genome project (HGP), who announced early in 2003, a complete mapping of the human genome. The findings of this genetic revolution will contribute to a greater understanding of human biology, and valuable new insights of disease causing pathogens that can all be applied to the control of diseases globally.

In many aspects, the work started in 1990 dubbed the human genome project continues unabated and current indicators are that future planned research undertakings for the human genome have no limits. Government policies have been established with available funding to sequence more than 2,300 complete human genomes, compared to only 34 by past findings. This, without doubt, has to contribute to research findings that will continue to benefit mankind.

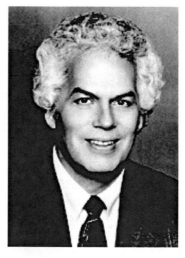

Stanley Ben Prusiner was born in Des Moines, Iowa, in 1942. After his secondary education, he attended the University of Pennsylvania where he received degrees in chemistry and medicine. Most of his professional career, to this day, has been at the University of California – San Francisco, where he became intrigued and challenged by the limited to no knowledge of the causation of the transmissible spongiform encephalopathies (TSEs). This concern became an affront to his professionalism and was amplified by the loss of one of his patients to Creutzfeldt-Jakob disease (CJD), a TSE disease, and the leading cause of death of sufferers of this complex group of encephalopathies in humans.

Answers as to cause – effect of the TSEs were needed, and he was intent to fully investigate the whys – with passion and resolve! Prusiner did investigate and research the whys of the spongiform encephalopathies, and, in the process, became part of medical history globally for his pioneering discovery of an entirely new theory of disease-causing agents that consisted entirely of protein that he gave the name, prion, abbreviated for "proteinaceous infectious particles." Prions exist normally in animals and man as cellular proteins, lack nucleic acid, are resistant to inactivation by physical and chemical treatments like irradiation, high temperatures, and enzymes that inactivate nucleic acid in conventional viruses and bacteria, tolerate a wide range of pH, between 2.5 and 10.5, long retention of infectivity for many months in 10 to 12 percent formalin, and triggers no immune response. Interestingly, prions are apparently not essential to life and their function in animals and man is unclear. Infectivity takes place when non-infectious cellular protein "folds" or converts to different conformations that trigger the genesis of pathogenic particles that result in lesion changes, particularly of neuronal tissues, and the ultimate progression to neurodegenerative signs of disease in animals and man that are always fatal.

The entire world of prion research, however, was shrouded with much initial criticism. The mere thought that a protein could be linked to pathology and fatal diseases was an affront to the fundamental concepts of disease causation, and many of Prusiner's doubters were unwilling to accept the theory. Skepticism prevailed. But, Prusiner, maintained a forward-looking and confident posture of assurance, supported by compelling research and published evidence that propelled his prion theory to acceptance in the mid-1990s. This was all taking place during a period of international debate about the TSEs in general, highlighted by the diagnosis of bovine spongiform encephalopathy (BSE), commonly referred to as "mad cow disease" in England in 1986.

This followed an interim assessment by animal health and public health officials in the United Kingdom, whether the newly identified disease in cattle had human health implications. During this early

122

phase of analyzing risk, the official thinking was that beef was likely safe and that the disease could not be transmitted by BSE-affected animals to people. This position changed quickly after the British government announced in March, 1996, that 10 young people had showed signs of a novel neurological disease, deemed a variant of CJD and "the most likely explanation for the cases of a new variant of CJD in young people was exposure to BSE." Research supported the analogy that the "misfolded protein extracted from the brains of both BSE-affected cattle and vCJD-affected human had an identical pattern that was different from the pattern seen in all other TSEs, including sporadic CJD."

The acute widespread uncertainty and trepidation involving the entire complexity of the public health relevance of the TSEs globally, and the cause, brought Prusiner to the epicenter of recognition, and the 1997 Nobel Prize in Physiology or Medicine for "the discovery of a new genre of disease-causing agents and the elucidation of their mode of action." While Prusiner's work has added prions to the world of infectious agents like bacteria, viruses, parasites and fungi, the overall significance has broader implications for the medical profession that could help examine the biological aspects/concepts of other neurodegenerative diseases like Alzheimer's and Parkinson's, and open vistas for control and treatment.

Prusiner remains a central figure in neurology throughout the globe, and with his cohorts at the University of California (San Francisco) and collaborators will likely add to the literature to the challenging field of degenerative diseases of the nervous system that affect both animals and man.

(B) The Disease Perspective
Infectious Diseases in Developed Countries

The general consensus based on assessments and determinants of health is that the health of the populations of the developed world in the last three decades has never been better. The influences of social, political and environmental factors helped to change the prevalence of disease patterns in different parts of the world. The supporting evidence was especially central to the decline of infectious diseases in developed countries that was responsible for an increase in life expectancy, but a greater incidence of the diseases commonly linked to aging populations like cancer, cardiovascular disease, arthritis, stroke, diabetes, obesity, mental diseases and depression, and other like diseases linked to the process of aging.

One very compelling reason why most of the developed and industrialized countries of the world have enjoyed this largesse of improved health is through the establishment of comprehensive health care programs for the people served. This is paid for and financed by varying forms of taxation and viewed as a public instrument for good governance, and the enhancement of public health. Interestingly, the United States where medical care has been market-driven, a transition by reform legislation is taking place and is time dependent how the change in policies will influence health. The debate is ongoing and passionate in scope with point – counter point and at times emotional political overtones. In fact, the comparatives of the United States to the rest of the world are difficult, if not impossible, because the 50 State governments of the country, unlike the rest of the world with predominantly nationally administered health programs, have the primary responsibility to protect public health on a State basis. Nonetheless, regardless of the system in place, there remains little doubt that the developed countries of the world, collectively, have well-organized and functional programs in place to control infectious diseases that have greatly contributed to the recognized improvements in health over the years, especially in the past two to three decades.

This, unfortunately, does not infer in any way, that the countries of the developed world are immune to the ravages and negative consequences of infectious diseases. Their long-term investments, however, in state of the art medical technology, the progress made in the provision of a clean water and a safe food supply, the importance and funding given to public health initiatives and research have contributed to the unprecedented gains made over the years. Just about every advanced society of the globe have instituted active and successful immunization programs, tuberculosis control programs, control and prevention programs for sexually transmitted diseases, including HIV/AIDS, ongoing infectious disease surveillance and education programs, and funding of disease control and prevention programs at academic and private sector settings. This constitutes a formidable infrastructure for the developed countries to respond to the challenges of infectious diseases, plus the available resources of good governance and management efficiency and a picture emerges.

The vulnerability of developed countries is linked to the emergence of infectious diseases that will mock infrastructure, ingenuity, resources, and governance, regardless of the attributes of these factors in disease surveillance, control and prevention practiced by industrialized countries. This is best exemplified by the HIV/AIDS complex. Several factors play a significant and important role that contributes to the new threats of the emerging infectious diseases, and while the developing countries are more prone to the variable risks, the developed countries are by no means immune. All countries experience in different degrees the problems associated with human demographics, behavior, susceptibility to infection, and the microbe-host interaction; genetic and biological forces that enhance mutation of microbes and regulation of genes for environmental adaptation; ecological factors like climate change and weather, and social, political, and economic factors like poverty, war and famine, inequality, and the breakdown of public health systems. Unfortunately, the developing countries continue to be challenged in a manner that remains so inequitable that progress seems undeniably evasive and limited, contributing to frustration, especially in the area of environmental degradation, economic development and use of land resources, lack of technology, climate and weather – typified by severe droughts and typhoons, behavior, education, poverty, lack of political advocacy, and the paucity of a public health tradition.

The aforementioned factors heighten the entire spectrum for the perpetuation of infectious diseases and a continuum that will threaten developed and developing countries, including the realization of the added burden for the resurgence of new antimicrobial resistant diseases. A successful response is dependent on a multidisciplinary approach – from epidemiological surveillance, diagnosis, to prevention and control strategies, and emergency responses when required. Developed countries, except in catastrophic circumstances, have the managerial capability and infrastructure for successful outcomes. Most, if not all, of the developing countries during an infectious disease crisis, need immediate assistance from the developed world. Realistically, the developing countries are still dependent on help and technical support in just about every facet of sustaining public health programs in their countries.

Infectious Diseases in Developing Countries

The continued characterization of developing countries as a generic term, while difficult to avoid, is downright unfortunate. It does not represent a realistic or true picture of the broad variables that exist between and within countries, and, as a result, complicate and distort issues to be analyzed fairly and objectively under the all-embracing banner of developing countries. Even some of the adjoining countries in sectors of the world like sub-Saharan Africa, Asia, Latin America and the Caribbean, the epicenter of some of our interests, are so obviously different, consideration must be given to assess a system for improved categorization of these countries to be better able to analyze with greater understanding and objectivity the problems that have to be addressed, even as we continue to treat the developing countries as an entity.

There is supporting data that suggests rapid changes, evidentiary of progress, have occurred in the health status of people living in some developing countries. The falling mortality rates in both infants and children, exemplified by improved immunization programs, are symptomatic of the success in controlling the prevalence of infectious diseases. An example is measles that causes widespread mortality in children because of concurrent infections like malaria and other forms of parasitism. This progress should be celebrated, but is still fraught with inequity in many of the least advanced countries that lack resources and a workable public health infrastructure. While children have been highlighted, the adult population also remains at risk, because an inadequate public health response system has no boundaries – every segment of the population, regardless of age, suffers from varying degrees of neglect related to access to basic primary health care services.

Some developing countries are still in a constant struggle for mere survival and infectious diseases like HIV/AIDS, tuberculosis, malaria, continue unabated, in spite of the yeoman efforts of many of their health professionals who reach out to the masses in spite of very limited resources. The sad realization is that while accepting that some progress is evident, the health systems in most of the developing countries will never be able to effectively deal with the existing deficiencies that impact needed improvements and responses to control and prevent infectious diseases. There is obvious immediacy and urgency for modifications and reform of health programs across the board in developing countries if there is going to be any hope to improve public health services for the most needy globally.

The majority of the developing countries remain an amalgam of needs – the need for clean water, safe food, improved sanitation and hygiene, better diagnostic capability, more doctors and support staff like technicians and nurses to treat the underserved, improved vaccination programs, more and less expensive medicines, better equipped clinics and hospitals, improved technology to serve needs, less bureaucratic controls, better disease surveillance, empowerment of the community, and a more interactive infrastructure for primary care and the control and prevention of infectious disease.

(C) Emerging Infectious Diseases: The Global Relevance

Newly diagnosed infections or old infections that have markedly increased in incidence or extended range of transmission geographically refer to the category of emerging infectious diseases. Fauci in a lecture in 2006 refined the concept of emerging into newly emerging diseases or those that have never been identified before; re-emerging or resurging as diseases that have been around for a long period of time but have returned in a different form or location e.g. West Nile virus from Africa to the United States; and, lastly, a new interesting category of deliberately emerging diseases associated with agents of bioterrorism e.g. the intentional introduction of the anthrax agent to cause harm to the public.

The causes of emerging diseases, with the exception of deliberately emerging, are associated with the genesis of an infectious agent into a new susceptible population, and the further capability of the agent to adequately adjust to the new environment and serve as a source of disease dissemination within the new population. A point of interest of global health concern is that approximately 75 percent of emerging infectious diseases are zoonotic and predominantly linked to wildlife origin. Additionally, the realization that there is compelling evidence based on research validation that HIV has an origin to zoonoses (cross species – animal to man transmission), amplifies the pertinence of the animal – human infection bond. In this specific viral transfer, HIV is considered the descendant of a Simian Immunodeficiency Virus (SIV) based on the resemblance of SIV to the two strains of HIV – HIV 1 and HIV 2 that infect humans. The most likely modes of infection between primates and man are consumption of "monkey" meat or bush meat or the blood of SIV-positive chimpanzees or monkeys getting into the cuts or wounds of hunters or others directly involved with varied forms of handling, either of the animals or the meat. This hypothesis has been widely accepted by the academic community, although other means of the initial transmission of the SIV virus to humans should not be overlooked. The thought, also, that HIV/AIDS, one of the most complex and challenging diseases in history, high morbidity and mortality, global ubiquity, and a defying affront to medicine and public health in the past three decades, could be linked with zoonotic implications, keep global public health in the realm of never ending uncertainty.

The fact that HIV/AIDS, comparatively, garnered the majority of the medical attention globally because of the aforementioned factors, it was only one of the approximately more than 30 new diseases that have been identified during the past three decades. Many of the newly described diseases are: Legionnaires' disease, hepatitis C, variant Creutzfeldt-Jakob disease linked to bovine spongiform encephalopathy, Nipah virus, hantavirus, Ebola virus/disease, Marburg disease, Rift Valley fever, monkey pox virus, severe acute respiratory syndrome (SARS), avian influenza virus (H5N1), Lyme disease and some hemorrhagic viral fevers. The anxiety and turmoil associated with the H1N1 (swine flu) virus in 2009 that challenged the health resources of about 20 or more countries in a short timeframe, heightens the importance of global vectors, their quick transmission potential, and their public health pertinence. Additionally, the resurgence of tuberculosis, cholera, and malaria adds the significance of the reemergence of infectious diseases, and the troubling dimensions to health, especially so in the developing countries, predominantly tropical, that provide a perfect climate and niche for the facilitation of threatening microbial vectors to transmit disease, most with zoonotic disease implications.

Discussion

Attempts to assess the diverse range of infectious diseases globally and their influence on health are challenging and frustrating, because of the impossible task to bring the broad spectrum of the subject into a semblance of coordinated and sequential information that is all embracing and representative. The history, itself, is so comprehensive that it has to be abridged to heighten major highlights, and, by design, limited to a period of time from the 1600s to the present, with the intent to capture nothing but the most influencing events that have had an indelible impact on the varied topics linked to infectious diseases.

A logical starting point was to recognize the role of the microscope in new discoveries of potential infectious agents, the development of early immunization strategies, aspects/concepts of infection control, experimentation and early research methods, the germ theory of disease, growth and innovations of diagnostic bacteriology, development and use of drugs and trials in chemotherapy, the identification of viruses in disease causation, the role of the mosquito as vectors of disease, the evolution of antibiotics to treat infections, genetics and mapping of the genome, to the characterization of prions – protein material – in the causative association of a broad range of neurodegenerative diseases of animals and man. These historical successes provide an insightful perspective of the continual progress made in the overall knowledge over centuries in infectious diseases, research, and medicine throughout the world, but markedly so in the developed countries, with resources and personnel dedicated to the advancement of science, and governments who support it.

The reaction and trend about sixty years ago, ironically, was optimism that the historical scourge of infectious diseases in the industrialized countries of the world was lessened by the introduction of improved public health programs, new and better vaccines and the promotion of immunization, the discovery and expansion of antibiotic use, a broad range of insecticides to control disease-causing vectors, heightened investigation and surveillance systems, and active disease control and prevention strategies. The latter part of the twentieth century mocked that feeling of ebullience. An inexplicable increase in the emergence and re-emergence of infectious diseases had started to take place in many parts of the world, and an interesting transformation in the association of microbe and man, likely due to ecological changes, migration, socio-economic factors, and changes in behavior were evident, affecting both the developed and developing countries. As previously implied, the developed countries have a built-in infrastructure to respond to threats of infectious diseases, while most developing countries, distressingly, are still in a constant struggle for mere survival, and the planned assaults on infectious diseases are not being realized.

The emerging and re-emerging infectious diseases, while problematic for all countries, are obviously especially so for the developing countries due to limited infrastructural response capabilities. Whether or not developing countries will ever be truly able to provide the anticipatory responses to the basic health needs of their populations, even in the midst of the increased prominence of health equity and social justice, remains an interesting unknown. There are, however, reasons for guarded optimism and hope. The influx of a new cadre of donors, contributing to new energy, direction, and a global vision with greater communicating linkages and cooperation between many developing countries, based on shared threats and challenges, contribute to the potential for positive change. This could help with long-term goals for building on national, regional and global health programs, using primary health care as part of a new collective movement for the control of infectious diseases, especially in resource poor countries. This will also support some of the thinking of the Millennium Development planners, by meeting the objectives of putting people at the center of the health care system, and the other needed improvements for disease control and prevention that includes an enhanced and sustained progressive public health agenda.

Conclusion

It is inconceivable to discuss the subject of infectious diseases without delving into some facets, albeit limited, of the contributors and contributions of history to the progress and success of the acquisition of knowledge of infectious diseases. Realistically, infectious diseases will most likely continue to play an important role throughout all countries of the globe, where we all need a collective and harmonized response to fight the diseases that plague us. The future will be most acute and contentious, however, for the developing countries that remain dependent on the global health network to increase their interventions to curtail the widespread problems of infectious diseases endemic to the global poor by investing in capacity building through greater financial commitments. This would complement the humanitarian outreach of developed countries, NGOs, and donors currently in place to marginalize poverty, and enable all people the potential to live more fulfilling and satisfying lives, and, in the process, build on both the socio-economic infrastructure and sustainable human development.

"Imagination should give wings to our thoughts, but we always need decisive experimental proof, and when the moment comes to draw conclusions and to interpret the gathered observations, imagination must be checked and documented by the factual results of the experiment."
Louis Pasteur, 1822-1895

"Public health is a bond – a trust – between a government and its people. The society at large entrusts its government to oversee and protect the collective good health. And in return individuals agree to cooperate by providing tax monies, accepting vaccines, and abiding by the rules and guidelines laid out by government public health leaders. If either side betrays that trust the system collapses like a house of cards."
Laurie Garrett
Betrayal of Trust: The Collapse of Global Public Health

Chapter 6

New Dimensions of Chronic Diseases

Introduction

In the last three decades, there is evidence of the emergence of a new phenomenon taking place throughout the developed world – people are living longer, and in many countries, the elderly are rapidly becoming the majority. This evolving transition over the years has been responsible for changing dimensions of disease prevalence and, specifically, the impact of aging and its importance to chronic diseases, including the treatment, control, and prevention of these diseases globally. As early as 1950, the population age group 65 years and older has increased from 8 percent to 13 percent. Indicators are that this trend will continue, and have become logical reasons for examining the new aspects and public health policies associated with and influencing this development. This overall pertinence of age-related diseases and the concurrent inferences for global public health programs in the future must be part of a new agenda. This trend, interestingly, does not appear to be limited to the most advanced countries, even some of the middle-income countries have started to witness this increased lifespan transformation in their societies. Aging worldwide, therefore, has to be taken into serious consideration in terms of both health policy prioritization and research in the future. Unfortunately,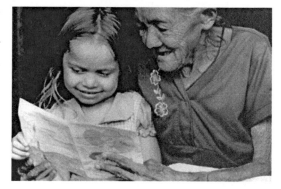

most of the developing countries do not possess the resources or technical and political commitment to make an impact that will address this transition.

While this demographic transition is comparatively recent, finite answers for the increased survival to older ages are predominantly speculative, but the logical assumption is that the overall improvements in public health, at least in the developed countries, must have contributed significantly. This is supported by findings that affirm the benefits of sanitation and hygiene, heightened by safe food and clean water, improved living conditions, increased access to immunization programs, and better medical interventions to be partially responsible. In like manner, lifestyle choices like diet, exercise, and cessation of smoking could have played contributory roles. Similarly, a poor diet with excessive fat intakes, overweight or obese states, lack of exercise or physical activity, smoking and excessive alcohol consumption could accelerate the rise in cardiovascular diseases, which remain the leading cause of death throughout the world, approximating nearly 18 million deaths annually. The longer life expectancy, therefore, comes with concurrent challenges – the need to address the increased population of elderly people in which cardiovascular diseases have become an epidemic and an affront to global public health.

In many developing countries, the rates of cardiovascular diseases are also on the increase due to greater affluence and a change in consumption habits and diets that parallel those of the developed countries. The intent is not to use cardiovascular diseases as an all-embracing metaphor for chronic diseases, but to highlight the relevance because of the prevalence and significance of this group of diseases globally. Worldwide, the total number of deaths for all causes approximate 58 – 60 million, of which chronic diseases will account for about 35-36 million. This is about double the number of deaths due to all infectious diseases (including HIV/AIDS, tuberculosis and malaria), and nutritional deficiencies combined. In reiterated amplification of the significance of cardiovascular diseases globally – about 18 million of the total chronic disease deaths are associated with that group of diseases. Additionally, the long-held misconception that chronic diseases is mainly a problem of high-income and affluent countries must be addressed – the fact is that 80 percent of the deaths in low and middle income countries are linked to chronic diseases. The realization and lesson learnt is that changes have evolved in the last three decades, and will likely continue along the same line in the future, in just about all countries of the globe, thus necessitating a new analysis of the entire spectrum of chronic diseases, and the need for prioritizing and adjusting to the new changing dimensions that will influence global health and policies, especially in resource-poor countries.

The Infectious Etiology of Chronic Diseases

As early as the 1800s, there was increasing suspicion in the global medical health community that many chronic diseases, including some forms of cancer, have an infectious disease origin. That thinking prevailed for many years, but did not meet the scientific validation or the "gold standard" of peer review acceptance. In the past three to four decades, however, there has been a convincing amount of cumulative data from different sectors of the world to link infectious agents to forms of cancer and other chronic diseases, some of which cause high morbidity and mortality, including cardiovascular disease, diabetes mellitus, and various neurological conditions.

Animal disease research has been a major contributing factor in the growth and development of medical knowledge over the centuries, thus, it was neither a surprise or unusual when centuries before viruses were fully defined and characterized as major causes of disease in humans, animals, and plants, there were anecdotal observations linking viruses to tumor formation in animals in the late 1800s. This observation provided researchers in human medicine to assess whether a same type of association exists in humans, opening up new vistas for comparative medicine and the benefits of animal models in the study of disease causation. The viral – neoplasm (tumor) linkages in animals were affirmed in both rabbits and poultry, exemplified by the Shope fibroma virus and infectious papillomas in domestic rabbits, and virus-induced tumors in poultry due to a herpesvirus known as Marek's disease, and the avian leucosis/sarcoma and reticuloendotheliosis caused by retroviruses. These early findings in animals were responsible, or at least set the stage, for more extensive research in the human study of oncology that could be linked to infectious agents. This transition heightened the value of collaborative research across the species barrier, and played an important role in today's emerging knowledge of a greater understanding of the etiology of tumors, their behavior, treatment, and possible control and prevention.

The infectious aspect of chronic diseases is well exemplified by a bacterium, Helicobacter pylori. This organism is likely the most widespread infection in the world, affecting about half of the world's population, and mostly linked to poor sanitation, fecal-oral transmission, and a compelling public health challenge in developing countries. H. pylori causes the two most common forms of peptic ulcer, chronic gastritis, and a small lifetime risk of gastric lymphoma, mucosa-associated lymphoid tissue (MALT) lymphoma, and gastric adenocarcinoma. Fortunately, infection can be mitigated and terminated by antibiotic therapy.

Cervical cancer, like most malignant neoplasms, is associated with a long latency and a multi-factorial etiology, but differs from other cancers as having as its major causal linkage - an infectious agent – the human papillomavirus (HPV). This proven relationship between a virus and cervical cancer has positive implications for public health and disease prevention through screening programs for HPV that will detect precursor lesions of cervical cancer. Commercially available HPV vaccines are in wide use in developed countries and highly recommended by public health officials for young women to prevent cervical cancer. HPV causes more than 90 percent of cervical cancers. The screening and vaccination programs would have a definite impact on the morbidity and mortality of cervical cancer, and a boost to public health globally. Unfortunately, the cost of the vaccine creates inequity and limited access in resource-poor countries whose inhabitants cannot afford the vaccine.

Lyme disease, named after the U.S. city of the same name in Connecticut in 1975, because of the initial clustering and diagnosis of the disease in the small town where it occurred. The disease is a tick-borne inflammatory disorder caused by Borrelia burgodorferi, an infectious spirochete. It is an illustrated example of how modifications in ecology and demographics can result in the emergence of new diseases – in this case, one that is vector-borne with complex symptoms varying from skin lesions due to the host's response to the tick bite, to late signs of neurologic, cardiac, and joint abnormalities (Lyme arthritis) developing as complex chronic manifestations.

The hepatitis B virus (HBV) accounts for more than 60 percent of liver cancers. The virus is transmitted through exposure to blood or blood-contaminated materials of infected persons. Evidence indicates that exposure leading to chronic infection occurs most frequently at birth when the mother is chronically infected with HBV, or in the first year of the newborn's life. In adults, epidemiologists at the Centers for Disease Control and Prevention in Atlanta, Georgia, have determined that the risks leading to exposure in the United States are sexual activity (about 50 percent of cases) and intravenous drug use (15 percent of cases).

These diseases were chosen because of their prevalence and impact on chronic disease epidemiology, treatment, prevention and control, and public health pertinence. There are also numerous examples of the microbe – chronic disease implications that deserve mentioning. There is research data that shows that infectious agents like, Chlamydia pneumoniae, may play a role in the pathogenesis of cardiovascular diseases like atherosclerosis, either as a primary pathogen or as a secondary contributing factor. This is important to disease control endeavors since atherosclerosis is a significant threat to global public health. The same infectious analogy applies to Campylobacter jejuni and Guillain-Barre syndrome, coxsackievirus to myocarditis, cytomegalovirus and varicella-zoster to congenital mental retardation, Chlamydia trachomatis to infertility, species of Schistosoma to urinary bladder and colonic carcinoma, enteroviruses to type 1 diabetes mellitus, and Japanese encephalitis virus to neuropsychiatric sequelae.

Many chronic disease specialists and researchers continue to follow the path for answers linking the causal relationship between infectious agents and chronic diseases. This new directional impetus of the association and suspected roles of microbes as primary or secondary contributors to a wide range of serious chronic diseases is an encouraging advance in the study of disease causation, diagnosis, and prevention that could help lessen the existing burden that chronic diseases impose globally., since there is a change in the nature of diseases attributed to infection. This advancement in knowledge could open new vistas for future research that will examine other causal linkages, and, in the process, assist the global efforts in the control and prevention, and treatment challenges of chronic diseases.

The Epidemiology of Chronic Diseases

The etiology and epidemiology of communicable diseases, especially when dealing with single-agent microbes like influenza, is comparatively easy to ascertain and control. The process is extremely more complicated with chronic diseases that are predominantly due to multiple causes. It is a daunting process to fully assess and determine with any degree of certainty the role of exposure hazards like poor sanitation and hygiene, malnutrition/hunger, excessive use of tobacco, environmental degradation, infectious agents and alcohol abuse, as single factors or cumulatively, influence the emergence of chronic diseases, and the impact on life expectancy and death, especially in developing countries, where surveillance and health assessments are seldom made due to limited resources and infrastructural deficits. This could also be a problem for many developed countries, because the

138

determinants of causation are complex, making the epidemiology of chronic diseases a heavy burden for research, necessitating long-term evaluations of the broad range of pathogenic mechanisms that warrant further investigations.

While accepting the many barriers and obvious limits that preclude a more insightful and informed analysis of the causation of chronic diseases, credit must be given to the rapid gains made in the last three decades in chronic disease epidemiology in developed countries, including the extensive amount of research data that has accumulated to determine prevalence of these diseases and strategies for prevention and control. In most countries of the world, including the United States, chronic diseases have become the leading cause of death and disability. According to the Centers for Disease Control and Prevention epidemiologists in the United States, chronic diseases account for 70 percent of the deaths – highlighted by heart disease, cancer, and stroke. About 50 percent of the country's adults had at least one chronic illness, with arthritis the most common cause of disability, and diabetes – the leading cause of kidney failure and other complications like blindness and amputations. Lung cancer remains the leading cause of cancer death with the vast majority of cases linked to cigarette smoking. Alcohol consumption and obesity are part of the varied risk factors that contribute to the burden of chronic disease epidemiology, especially in the developed countries, but an emerging concern in middle income societies, mimicking the lifestyle/behavior of developed countries.

Global mortality comparisons of chronic diseases and their implications for both developed and developing countries are interesting. It is important that many of the middle and low income countries take a signal for action from the developed countries and recognize the importance of chronic diseases and the mandate for a new approach for prevention and control efforts. The fact that 80 percent of deaths attributable to chronic diseases occur in middle and low income countries should be the cue for a renaissance. The global risk associated with about 1 billion people being overweight, and 2.6 million dying of linkages to that "pathology" highlights the challenge. Current projections that about 388 million people will likely succumb to a chronic disease in the next 10 years, amplifies the overall public health dilemma. There is, nonetheless, cause for optimism if a concerted global response is put in place. Health officials have fully identified the major causes and risk factors contributing to morbidity and mortality of chronic diseases globally. Elimination of the risk-associated factors could prevent about 80 percent of deaths caused by heart disease, stroke, and type 2-diabetes, and over 40 percent of cancer.

The prevailing consensus that CVD is a disease of affluence, albeit true, and is especially problematic for industrialized societies whose populations consume and indulge in unhealthy diets, must be debated. The subject was detailed in an impressive publication by Beaglehole and Yach in the Lancet in 2003. The authors claim that 80 percent of CVD deaths occur in low and middle income countries, supplemented by findings using mortality data from China and India that twice as many deaths from CVD occur in less developed countries than developed countries. Additionally, CVD is responsible for about 2.8 million deaths in China, and 2.5 million deaths in India annually, providing a perspective of the immense problem the developing countries face with the prevalence of chronic diseases, exemplified by the two most populous countries on earth. Interestingly, while CVD mortality has shown impressive declines in just about all the developed countries, the resource-poor countries continue to experience rapid increases in their mortality rate.

Estimates of the approximate number of cancer cases worldwide is about 10 million, with the incidence in men somewhat higher than in women, accounting for about 7 million deaths annually. The disease also has a greater incidence in developing countries, over five million, compared to approximately 4.7 million for developed countries. The most common malignant neoplasms reported in men were lung, stomach, colorectal, prostate and liver; while in women, breast, colorectal, cervical, lung, and ovarian were the most frequent. The major predisposing causes of cancer in all countries were tobacco use, chronic infections in developing countries, and a complicated and ill-defined mixture of dietary, environmental, and other factors.

Tobacco remains the principal cause of cancer worldwide – its use is directly responsible for the high incidence of lung cancer, the most common occurring cancer globally, causing approximately 30 percent of all human cases, including cancers of the larynx, oral cavity, pharynx, esophagus, pancreas, kidney, and bladder. The convincing research findings over the years linking use of tobacco to cancer, has resulted in an impressive decline in smoking in many developed countries that would likely result in a decreased incidence in lung and other cancers in the future. Regulations in most developed countries (and some developing countries) limiting smoking in restaurants, offices, public buildings, airports, and litigations over the years against the tobacco companies, for example, the United States, have increased public consciousness of the dangers and hazards to health. Unfortunately, this is not taking place with the same intensity in most developing countries where cancer caused by smoking tobacco is increasing with a concurrent spiraling of deaths. The World Health Organization published data to indicate that about 100,000 children start smoking around the world every day, and about a third of the adult male population has acquired the habit, contributing to the sale of 15 billion cigarettes every day. That number equates to about three cigarettes a day for every human on the planet.

Chronic respiratory diseases include (a) chronic obstructive pulmonary disease (COPD), comprising chronic bronchitis, emphysema, bronchiectasis, bronchial catarrh, and other non-specific airway diseases; and (b) asthma. They are collectively significant causes of morbidity and mortality in developing countries accounting for 4.8 percent of mortality worldwide. Most of the deaths due to COPD occur in China and India, accounting for more than two-thirds of mortalities because of the continuing excessive use of tobacco, air pollution (indoors and outdoors), environmental and occupational factors, and the occurrence of respiratory infections early in life.

While asthma deaths are rare globally, they could occur. The main public health concern with asthma is the wide prevalence and morbidity, in both industrialized and resource-poor countries. Many of the risk factors are the same associated with COPD, but additional potential sources like dust and allergens could trigger asthmatic attacks.

Tuberculosis continues to be a challenging dilemma, especially troubling for public health officials in developing countries. The thought that someone in the world dies of tuberculosis every 18 seconds should be cause for unceasing contemplation. The disease is a core component in the annals and study of infectious diseases, having a millennia long history, and a cause of death in humans for at least 3,000 years. Sadly, it is not a disease of the past, but a continuing threat to the globe due to indifference, complacency, and a lack of commitment by many countries to keep prevention and control initiatives as priorities in their public health strategies. Unfortunately, in most of the least developed countries with the highest incidence of tuberculosis, and where survival from day to day is the norm, the needed infrastructural response to have an impact does not exist. This disease is one of the prime examples of the pathology of poverty.

Tuberculosis is a perfect illustration of health inequity, when one

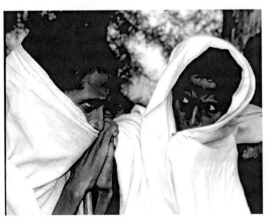

considers that about 95 percent of those infected live in developing countries, with Africa and Asia, the most affected regions. To confound and complicate the global picture and public health challenge, the disease has formed an "alliance" with

142

HIV/AIDS that accelerates the progression of the disease, and an increase in mortality. The global estimates of some epidemiologists working with HIV/AIDS are that about one-third of deaths are due to co-infection with tuberculosis, especially in areas of sub-Saharan Africa.

The problem of drug-resistant tuberculosis is worldwide, and particularly problematic in developing countries due to "poor clinical practice, inadequate supervision and resources, and unethical commercial sales of anti-tuberculosis drugs and combinations." Inadequate or incomplete treatment of the disease has been responsible for the development of new resistant strains to the drug armament that previously destroyed the causative organism in 100 percent of cases, creating what some infectious disease specialists describe as the "third epidemic," and an uphill battle for treatment and control efforts of tuberculosis globally.

Diabetes mellitus is expected to be a continuing challenge to global health. It has been estimated that the incidence of this condition worldwide is about five percent, based on findings in 2003, but chronic disease epidemiologists are projecting a steady increase in the prevalence of this disease over the next 25 years, mostly in developing countries. These estimates can be directly correlated to reduction in physical activity and dietary changes that have taken place in the past three decades. Interestingly, researchers have estimated based on current trends that by the year 2025, over 70 percent of the 300 million suffering from diabetes worldwide will be living in the less developed countries. A comparative to the United States illuminates the dilemma. In fact, diabetes mellitus is "the fourth most common reason for patient contact with a physician and is a major cause of premature disability and mortality. It is the leading cause of blindness among working-age people, of end-stage renal disease, and of non-traumatic limb amputations."

Chronic Diseases: Impact on Developing Countries – Global Health Relevance

Chronic diseases remain a defying challenge to global health, exemplified by what is dubbed diseases of affluence – cardiovascular diseases, cancer, and diabetes, and a need for corrective programs worldwide. Fortunately, comparisons are not difficult to make. The developed countries have well-defined goals and an infrastructure to respond, while the developing countries, for the most part, continue to depend on external sources of assistance to address the varying threats to health that contribute directly or indirectly to the excess prevalence of chronic diseases. The external donors or sources contributing to aid are mainly geared for the plight of those living in the 90 or so least developed countries. This could also vary and generally lack the permanence that is necessary, or funding, to foster a meaningful agenda for change. In the majority of interventions, the central focus is responding to the most pressing health problems, which are often temporary in scope, and never enough to meet the urgent demands of a community or country long-term.

Equally problematic, many of the responses are linked to acute emergencies and disease outbreaks of an infectious nature, often with high morbidity and mortality, like cholera, but never really programmed to strategically respond to the nuances of chronic diseases, and the complex underlying causes that will create progress to ensure change. We continue to live with the barriers of development – a poor government = poor resources = poor services = poor health care = malnutrition/hunger = disease – hopelessness = and the obvious need for social justice to correct the inequities. Millions around the world still die each day, simply because they are too poor to stay alive. The problem transcends health and disease, and should be programmed to establish a workable system to effectively reduce the burden of sickness and death inequalities suffered by the poor and destitute of the world.

The goals instituted by developed countries for health promotion – disease surveillance and response, capacity building, prevention and control programs, research and education, structure and infrastructure – are lacking in developing countries. This illustrates the vast existing differences and disparities between the countries that have resources and those that do not. It is also impossible to expect countries with a per capita income of $1 or less a day to program chronic disease surveillance, prevention, and capacity building when they cannot maintain a supply of clean water, or the other elementary sanitary and hygienic necessities that contribute to health, and, hopefully, mitigate the emergence of chronic diseases. The circumstances mock reality. The people in most of the less developed countries are most concerned about surviving another day and obtaining something to eat than far-reaching programs to promote health and control disease. Many have little confidence that proposed improvements could be made to truly address their plight and concerns, at least in a sustained and meaningful manner. That is inherent in the hopelessness factor that is so prevalent in nearly all of the developing countries. It defies a definition. It is a mixture of faith, hope, and charity! It is simply something that is felt through the experience of life and living under adverse conditions. Today, often looks so much like yesterday in most developing countries – very little or nothing to eat, and tomorrow will not be much better, and could likely be worse. The cycle is predictable and constant – very few jobs to contribute to the well-being of a family and little hope that the situation will change in the foreseeable future.

The difficult to answer challenge continues – how to control diseases in societies that lack the elementary resources to do so. In the developing countries where life and living is burdened by extreme poverty, and the prevalence of complex tropical diseases, and many national governments unable to identify the major determinants for maintaining health, the future is formidable. The interim reaction to this impasse is treat existing diseases, with prevention and control playing a secondary role due to sparse or no resources. Some of the most influential forces of health and disease control are beyond the control of public health authorities, and include the general conditions of living – lack of sustainable agriculture and food production, housing, employment, education, and economic ventures to heighten equity. Chronic diseases are only one part of the cumulative problems in the totality of challenges that

145

have to be prioritized in most developing countries without the resources or leadership to do so.

In developing countries, people do not have access, or cannot afford, the diagnostic tests for the early detection of chronic diseases like diabetes or cancer. Even if they did, it is not customary for them to seek these services for varied reasons, other than access or cost. Thus, many of these diseases are diagnosed at an advanced stage, complicating treatment and increasing the likelihood of death. Many people, some elderly, in developing countries, have never been examined by a doctor and often seek medical help as a last resort and during life threatening circumstances. There is widespread neglect and indifference relating to chronic disease programs due to poor advocacy and limited resources for long-term strategic agendas to have an impact.

No generic guidelines will ever apply that could meet the objectives of chronic disease prevention and control in resource-poor countries. Conditions and needs vary to such a marked degree from country to country that initiatives could only succeed based on individualized assessments of countries. Many lives continue to be marginalized and lost because there are often no treatment facilities for effective long-term care and management of chronic diseases, even when the interventions are workable and inexpensive. Risk reduction strategies could be promoted through educational programs by maximizing and optimizing the use of government-private sector alliances at minimal costs, for example, at community meetings or work places. The promotion of vaccination programs for the prevention of cervical cancer, a major cause of mortality in developing countries, could start at schools. This approach could save millions of lives over the years. The availability of drugs to treat HIV/AIDS, tuberculosis, and malaria at an affordable price and with government and pharmaceutical industry support will go a long way to mitigate disease prevalence of these three killer diseases. A program to assure medication compliance could heighten the success.

Don A. Franco

The cost of drugs and medicines in developing countries prevents the majority of inhabitants from enjoying the benefits of treatment and becomes a serious deterrent that has to be addressed by health authorities and the political establishment. This is not limited to HIV/AIDS, tuberculosis, and malaria, but just about all the chronic diseases that need treating over a prolonged period of time like diabetes, cardiovascular disease, and some treatable cancers. The pathology of poverty makes no exceptions. It embraces every aspect of life. Education must be factored into the correctives to help people's awareness about the broad role of public health, including safe sex, and the other practices and behaviors that will help prevent diseases, infectious and chronic. This should start at school and could hopefully serve as a basic introduction to health fundamentals that could contribute to long-term awareness and the involvement of the community at large.

Access to clinics and hospitals in many developing countries is a difficult undertaking, and even when accessible, the services available or provided might not meet the needs of the patients. This is heightened by lengthy waiting periods under challenging conditions, crowding, and bureaucratic procedures that contribute to no encouragement to return and utter frustration. This is often compounded by the understaffing of health care facilities, making it necessary for patients to return for services at a later date. This is inherent to most health care systems in developing countries and is accepted by the populations served, because options do not exist. Choice is only a dream, and hope eternal. In many regions of the world there is simply no choice. There is also no program to identify those who are most in need of medical services and at risk, including the old and disabled, and the mentally impaired. The immediate family becomes the only available resource in most cases.

The treatment, management, prevention and control of chronic diseases remain complex without ready solutions. Developing countries will continue to be stressed because of limited resources, infrastructural deficits, poor governance, and lack of direction and commitment. Developing partnerships within the country with

147

NGOs, and representatives of international donors and foundations to pursue objectives will help. The ultimate progress and success, however, will depend on the correction of the predisposing causes – the greatest of which is poverty. If poverty is not marginalized and alleviated in a manner to help economic growth and development, resource poor countries will continue to experience the indignities of impoverishment, hunger, and disease. In fact, we have been saying these things for years, and while some improvements have been apparent, the global situation for chronic disease management and control has a long way to go, if we truly plan to provide semblances of hope to those who are currently hopeless. Health programs, to be truly effective and sustainable, must be delivered concurrently with other socio-economic pursuits of countries.

Discussion/Conclusion

The nuances and new dimensions of the changing world of chronic diseases, including the new information and knowledge in the past three decades, demand a renaissance type of approach. The fact that people are living longer throughout the world, with the exception of countries in sub-Saharan Africa where HIV/AIDS has altered that trend in life expectancy, affirms the new challenges that have evolved, and the creation of a new era for the study, prevention, and control of chronic diseases. The longer life expectancy globally necessitates the need for a reevaluation of the changing conditions and circumstances of life to respond to these new dimensions with a new resolve, and broad collaboration with the medical research community in every region of the world. The contracted globe provides ample opportunities for joint research endeavors and cooperation to benefit mankind and disease control. The developed and developing worlds have historically learnt from joint ventures over the years, and this togetherness must continue.

The new affirmation that infectious agents have an association with chronic diseases helps to expand the world of epidemiology and provides impetus to fully investigate the role of microbes in chronic

148

Don A. Franco

diseases including cancer. Optimism is a natural response when the possibility to conquer the high mortality caused by cervical cancer, especially in developing countries, is realized through early immunization. This introduction of an effective commercial vaccine can save millions of lives over the years. The same can apply to other viral agents like HBV linked to liver cancer and a source of widespread mortality globally. This is surely a new beginning for chronic disease ventures, and a source of excitement of the many unknowns that potentially exist and need revelation.

Many daunting challenges remain. The exposure hazards, singly or cumulatively, like the use of tobacco, a major contributing cause of various forms of cancer, must become a major objective for global public health research. Both the morbidity and mortality linked to smoking must be amplified as prioritized objectives, exemplified by China and India, where the problem remains defiantly overwhelming, and a burden to these two countries public health systems, comprising one third of the world's population. All the future epidemiological indicators show the prevalence of chronic diseases will increase, especially in the developing countries, many with limited or no resources to circumvent either the current of future challenges for prevention and control.

The obvious variables between the developed countries that have the necessary resources and the developing countries that have not will continue to be problematic for the control of chronic diseases. The developed countries with a health infrastructure that has the capability to adjust to change and make modifications when needed contrast sharply with the poor countries that lack resources for developing or maintaining what are already in place – this disparity will perpetuate inequities and contribute to a lack of programs that could impact prevention and control initiatives. The fact is that resource-poor governments simply cannot build the responses needed to guarantee their citizens any hope for lasting or sustainable services. The idea that any "gold standard" of health could be developed or sustained in countries where many of the inhabitants live on less than $1 a day is ludicrous. What can governments in

149

developing countries, especially the lowest income countries, do to change this inequity? Is there really hope in this forest of abject hopelessness? And, where do we begin to institute programs that will make a difference in the lives of the affected people? How do we truly do the things needed to influence change? Will the burden of chronic diseases continue indefinitely, or is there a global health program that will lift the poverty-stricken from the doldrums of nothingness?

The situation is never simple when dealing with the diverse complexities that challenge the less developed countries. It is more than just poverty and the prevalence of chronic diseases, regardless of their relevance or importance. It is also about the role of governance, infrastructure, and environmental degradation contributing to disease causation. It is about limited independence and the frustrating reality of being nothing more than recipients from donor countries, at times, for resources, for mere survival. That dependence has a price. It is about misuse of scarce resources, and the inability to prioritize needs and plan with sustained objectivity to develop programs to assist people in dire need to move forward. It is about motivation and good leadership. It is about providing hope in an atmosphere of hopelessness. Fortunately, many good people throughout the world including donor governments and international NGOs and foundations, are fully understanding of the acute needs of the least developed countries, and are working collaboratively to correct the existing burdens, in spite of some of the many frustrations that become barriers to their efforts and resolve.

One would have to be totally indifferent not to be truly sympathetic to the plight of the many in need during a period when so much is available. But, the developing countries must continue with their own progressive agenda to help themselves become fully independent, without which, countries can never be truly free. While there is no evidence of that happening any time soon, the collective force of humanism and benevolence should keep us optimistic that we are all in this together and must cooperate and collaborate together for the greater benefit of all. The thought that 60 to 75 percent of people in developing countries still lack access to basic primary health care is unacceptable if we have any hope for health programs to be effective and sustainable and part of social and economic development globally. The problem continues to be very basic – what must we do to make life and living more comfortable for the poor of our planet? And, what can we do collectively to treat, prevent, and control chronic diseases from being the overwhelming burden that it is today, and, will likely continue to be in the future.

"Healthy people are those who live in healthy homes on a healthy diet in an environment equally fit for birth, growth, work, healing, and dying."
John Illich, 1926-

"People are the driving force behind development, and a future of peace, progress, and stability depends on giving priority to the needs and rights of all people. Whatever the efforts and resources that must be invested in this enterprise, they will be small compared with the riches that a healthy and productive population represents."
Carlyle Guerra de Macedo, 1937-

Chapter 7

Hunger and Malnutrition

Introduction

Humans need a food source to supply energy and the nutrients that are essential for life, growth, and reproduction. Nutrition is more than a balanced diet and the efforts to achieve in diets what are considered "recommended levels" of nutrients. The subject is complex and a part of clinical medicine, linked to diverse disease conditions like diabetes mellitus, coronary heart disease, and cancer, and a major force in global public health.

Before delving into the subject of hunger and malnutrition, the entire assessment of food production, sustainable agriculture, globalization, policies and politics of world trade, and the force of economics must be 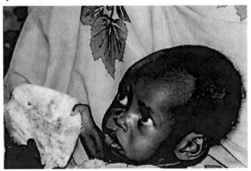 considered prior to addressing the broad nuances of hunger and malnutrition with emphasis on developing countries. In most (if not all) resource-poor countries, a general improvement in food production is necessary to boost economic growth and development, particularly in the rural areas, the epicenter of agricultural activity. This has to evolve through national governments' investments in agriculture and treating farming initiatives as priorities in a country's overall development plan with well-defined short-term and long-term objectives; properly implemented, the result could be enhanced prosperity to the rural community, an improved standard of living and heightened equity. The objectives, to be successful, however, must be supplemented by research and active collaboration with the agricultural community to pursue goals that would adapt best to the stressed environments, including limited land and water resources of the less developed countries.

Policies must also be promoted to give farmers the necessary incentives to move beyond the limitations of mere subsistence, and governments must serve as active catalysts, working in harmonization with the farming communities, to ascertain forward-looking programs to improve yields, both crops and livestock, become a central focus of a progressive agenda that can be sustained. Without government's involvement and support of the agricultural development toward sustainability, little progress will be ever realized in conquering the blight and despair of hunger and malnutrition. In fact, food production and the success of it is a joint responsibility (and accountability) of the government and the people who produce the food, and only by working in unison with a programmed agenda could improvements take place. No one group working independently can do it alone. The challenges are too complex for any form of individualism, and nothing short of a collective and organized venture will suffice.

Hunger is by no means a new affliction of mankind. The subject has been discussed and a feature of history throughout civilization, and amplified by biblical references and early religious texts. In fact, the scarcity of food has been debated for millennia, yet, continues to be an unnecessary and widespread challenge in the 21st century in a world with the resources to feed everyone on earth. It is complex and a failure of basic capabilities. Its persistence in spite of the dramatic technological advances in food production globally in the past fifty years should be deemed scandalous and unacceptable. The word, hunger, has different meanings, but the underlying link is related to the uneasy sensation and exhausted condition caused by want of food, or a signal that the body wants to or needs to eat. In the context of this book, hunger will be highlighted as the want or scarcity of food in a country or throughout the world as applicable. There are very few social or economic challenges facing the world today that are more pressing than hunger, and the consequences of it, especially in the developing countries of Asia and Africa.

Malnutrition is indicative of a lack of some or all nutritional elements needed for health. This deficiency can be considered from two perspectives – protein-energy malnutrition (PEM), which is a lack of sufficient protein and food to provide energy, a serious challenge in all resource-poor countries, and a reflection of the hunger index, to a degree. The other form of malnutrition is a deficiency of vitamins and minerals or micronutrient malnutrition. PEM, globally, is the most problematic form of malnutrition/hunger worldwide.

Hunger and malnutrition, however, is not a simple issue, and transcends the mere production of more food as a magical solution. While increased food production would serve as a definite improvement, the reality is that the overall complexity of hunger and malnutrition overlaps into all spheres of society and will continue to mock and defy the efforts of decision makers in developing countries, unless the correctives embrace the pre-disposing factors that are contributory. Good motives have proven not to be a remedy. And, poverty, the most challenging negative for growth and a semblance of equity, including the marginalization of hunger and malnutrition, seems beyond the current capability of existing global institutions. It should be of interest to those with a world view to realize that the hunger-malnutrition alleviation has been "tackled" previously by ideal motives, exemplified by the World Food Conference in Rome in 1974 with the proposal to eliminate hunger within a decade. The totality of the challenge seems beyond the comprehension of those who establish policy dictates. The current debates globally exemplify how elusive the correctives for hunger and malnutrition are when assessments of the points – counter points are made. In fact, the lesson could be – we just do not realize the extent of the challenge or what is necessary to correct it!

Since the association of poverty to hunger and malnutrition are so interrelated, attempts to separate the bonds would be circumventing the obvious. The failure remains very basic – the global political infrastructure's inability to establish systems to assist people in the developing countries maintain the needed strategic plans to produce enough food in a sustainable manner to meet the minimum nutritional requirements for energy to help alleviate hunger and malnutrition. While it is comparatively easy to identify this basic failure, one would be blindly naïve to think that ready solutions would emerge to correct the disparity. The problem is so deeply ingrained in man's history that the reality of it persisting to defy our collective ingenuity remains the challenge.

Mortality due to hunger/malnutrition accounted for about 58 percent of total deaths, in which more than 36 million died of hunger or deficiency diseases linked to malnutrition in 2006. The World Health Organization has published data to show that malnutrition has a direct or indirect association with about half of all cases of child mortality worldwide. Children who are malnourished grow up with more health problems and achieve less educationally than the well-nourished. Malnutrition has also been proven to exacerbate complications with many infectious diseases in children like measles, pneumonia, and diarrhea, and increases the risk of the onset of tuberculosis.

A person dies on average every second of causes linked to malnutrition – 100,000 each day. About every 5 seconds, a child dies of malnutrition or about 16,000 daily, accounting for about 60 percent of all child deaths. While childhood malnutrition is an integral part of life in developing countries, it is also an ongoing challenge in developed countries like the United States where over 3 million children under 5 years of age are at risk of hunger. And, while no one really knows the exact number of people who are hungry or malnourished, we remain dependent on the United Nations Food and Agriculture Organization that performs the measures. Their estimates indicate a depressing increase in hunger/malnutrition globally due to lack of agricultural development and food production in developing countries, the current global economic crisis, and a significant increase in food prices that especially impact the resource-poor countries.

Nutritional Deficiencies –
(Emphasis - Protein-energy Malnutrition)

Malnutrition is an all-embracing term covering any form of nutritional disorder of an individual (or groups of people), so both obesity and starvation, representing opposite spectra are technically included. The condition is rarely linked to a single nutrient, and in developing countries, malnutrition often manifests as a non-descript clinical syndrome with varied symptoms that are usually associated with a deficiency of several nutrients. These ill-defined symptoms make a specific diagnosis impossible, because of the multiplicity of the clinical signs. The long-held fallacious perception that posits the only or main cause of malnutrition is not consuming needed nutrients through a proper diet, overlook the syndrome observed in most developing countries, and some of the other elusive elements in play. Malnutrition and hunger overlaps with poverty, environmental degradation, infectious diseases with concomitant parasitism, poor dietary habits, civil war conflicts and famine, especially in regions of sub-Saharan Africa and Asia.

Malnutrition can be divided into two main categories: primary, associated with a failure to eat proper foods, and secondary, a result of an increase in requirements, metabolic disorders, and a decrease in absorption or an increase in excretion. In essence, a broad range of factors are linked to secondary malnutrition which often occurs as complications of other conditions, including many underlying diseases.

Three forms of protein-energy malnutrition (PEM) remain distinct threats to at risk populations in developing countries: marasmus, kwashiorkor (KW) and marasmic kwashiorkor (KW). These protein deficiencies are seen in the less developed countries, in children with nutritional and energy deficits, at the time of weaning or post-weaning. Marasmus is a serious global health problem that afflicts more than 50 million children less than five years old. PEM is a defying problem killing millions of children in developing countries annually. Children from countries that enjoy a good standard of living are also affected, especially those living in large urban areas, those at the low end of the economic ladder, or those who are institutionalized or suffer from chronic diseases. Therefore, the underprivileged, even in advanced or industrialized countries are at risk dependent on their circumstances.

Marasmus refers to the specific state where both calorie and protein intakes are severely limited and is an adaptive response to an insufficient energy intake. This energy deficit is accompanied by a decrease in physical activity, lethargy, weight loss – characterized by marked muscle wasting and loss of subcutaneous fat – and associated growth retardation with a pronounced loss of electrolytes, minerals, and vitamins. Marasmus is accompanied by immune impairment and infections.

Globally, nearly 30 percent of humans experience one or more of the multiple forms of malnutrition with a concurrent heavy toll on morbidity and mortality. Approximately 70 million people show varied signs of wasting and another 230 million or so different degrees of stunting. Estimates have clearly determined the regions of the world that are most at risk – 50 percent of Asian children, 30 percent of African, and 20 percent of Latin American are undernourished. This demographic profile corresponds predictably to the published epidemiology of malnutrition based on population dynamics and prevailing poverty in the different regions of the world.

Kwashiorkor, in contrast to marasmus, is a deficit caused by inadequate protein intake while a fair to good energy (total calories) intake is present. Like any condition associated with malnutrition, kwashiorkor manifests early in life with the general signs of fatigue and lethargy, with many of the affected children being easily irritated. As the condition progresses, clinical symptoms can include the loss of muscle mass, minimal growth, edema in the form of generalized swelling with a protruding abdomen, thinning and reddish discoloration of the hair, skin conditions with changes in pigmentation ("flaky paint" dermatosis), and in the later stages of the disease, a child's face appears to what some clinicians describe as a "bulldog" face. The symptoms in the terminal phase of kwashiorkor are shock and coma. The condition has its descriptive origin from one of the Kwa languages of Ghana, meaning "the one who is displaced," since it is mostly seen in weaned children that have to be breastfed.

Marasmic KW, reflects the name. It is a mixed form of PEM. It manifests clinically as both wasting and edema, in contrast to marasmus that is typified by wasting, and kwashiorkor in which the main sign is edema.

Major Deficiency Diseases

An introduction of the major deficiency diseases is a mere micro-overview to highlight the pertinence of these diseases to hunger and malnutrition and the concomitant impact of these deficiencies to the inhabitants of developing countries – the most affected and at risk populations.

Vitamin A deficiency (VAD) (xenopthalmia) is most often seen in severely malnourished children in developing countries. In its most extreme manifestation, this deficiency could lead to blindness. The condition remains a serious public health problem among the poor and undernourished in resource-poor countries and can be treated or prevented by adequate diets or fortification with foods rich in vitamin A like fish oils, beef, liver and egg yolk. Globally VAD is a clinical or subclinical problem in about 80 of the world's countries, mainly in Southeast Asia and sub-Saharan Africa with an estimated 250 million children at risk. VAD data is not precise, because accurate information is difficult to compile in resource-poor countries where the deficiency is most rampant. Nonetheless, assessments from public health organizations indicate about a quarter to a half million children become blind annually due to VAD.

Don A. Franco

The major biological function of vitamin D is the maintenance of normal blood levels of calcium and phosphorus. Rickets in children is a prime example of a vitamin D deficiency manifesting during the first two years of life, later becoming a chronic disorder of the young, contributing to skeletal deformities like bowed legs and knock-knees in the malnourished. The deficiency is seldom seen in developed countries due to a high standard of living and adequate diets, but does occur in the poverty stricken of these countries due to poor nutrition, a lack of exposure to the sun, or a syndrome in which the intestines fail to absorb nutrients from the food. In adults, the deficiency, defined as osteomalacia, is associated with muscular weakness and "weak" bones.

Vitamin B1 or thiamine is found in many foods like cereal grains, nuts, beans, yeast and meat, and is necessary for carbohydrate metabolism. A deficiency can produce neurological, cardiac, and gastrointestinal symptoms, depending on the degree of the deficiency. Asians are prone to this deficiency because their diets consist mainly of polished rice in which the husk that contains the vitamin is lost during the polishing process. In some regions of the world this could result in a severe form of beriberi characterized by nerve, brain, and heart abnormalities. The nerve condition, known as dry beriberi, manifests as pin-like sensations in the toes with a burning feeling in the feet at night, accompanied by muscle cramps and pain. Brain or cerebral beriberi is due to a sudden and severe deficit of thiamine associated with mental confusion and double vision at times. This syndrome, if not properly treated, could result in coma and death. The heart abnormalities or wet beriberi are typified by shortness of breath, dizziness, and irregularities in the heart beat. An interesting acute infantile beriberi occurs in babies who are breast-fed by thiamine deficient mothers. This condition could result in cardiac failure and death of infants if not treated promptly and properly.

Vitamin B2 or riboflavin is needed by the body to use oxygen and to metabolize amino and fatty acids, carbohydrates, and is required for the health of mucous membranes of the digestive tract.

159

A deficiency (ariboflavinosis) is uncommon in developed countries. It is similar to thiamine from a causal association because it is mainly seen in regions of the world where polished rice predominates in the diet. Symptoms of this deficiency are characterized by oral lesions (sores in the corners of the mouth and cracks in the lips), dermal lesions, mostly of the genitalia, and ocular lesions that vary from an interstitial keratitis to corneal opacity.

Niacin is also known as nicotinic acid, vitamin PP, and vitamin B3, because it was the third of the B vitamins to be discovered. It is found in a variety of animal products like chicken, beef, fish, milk and eggs, and fruits and vegetables like avocados, tomatoes, broccoli, dates, and carrots. Like most other nutritional deficiencies, a deficiency is rarely seen in industrialized countries, other than those living in poverty and malnourished. A severe deficiency of niacin in the diet causes pellagra (derived from the Italian word for rough skin), characterized by dermatitis, especially of the arms and legs, diarrhea, dementia, "necklace" lesions of the lower neck, inflammation of the mouth and tongue, digestive disturbances, and death if not properly treated.

Niacin deficiency is also seen concurrent with a deficiency of tryptophan, an amino acid which is needed in its synthesis. This deficiency is typical of the other deficiency diseases in poor countries due to a mixture of limited diets linked to the constraints caused by poverty and the restricted availability of foods. In the case of pellagra, considered a pandemic deficiency disease, the major prevalence occurs in countries of the world where maize (corn) is the principal food cereal. Unfortunately, maize has a low content of tryptophan and much of the niacin is in a bound form. In some African and Asian countries where sorghum or millet is the main cereal in the diet, pellagra is also a public health challenge.

Iron is an essential mineral needed by the body, and is a part of all cells, exemplified by the protein, hemoglobin, that carries oxygen from the lungs throughout the body. Iron deficiency is due to too little iron in the body, and the leading cause of iron deficiency anemia, likely the most common nutritional deficiency in the world.

Due to the high standard of living and the availability of a diverse food supply rich in iron (meat, fish, poultry), iron deficiency is seldom seen as a nutritional disease in developed countries, except in a limited number of vegetarians, or some with individual food idiosyncrasies or consumption habits. In developing countries, however, iron deficiency anemia remains a continuing challenge in school age children affecting more than half due to inadequate diet and a low intake of food rich in iron, often combined with infection, particularly hookworm and malaria. Blood loss is an important factor throughout the tropical world due to the prevalence of intestinal parasites like hookworms affecting over 700 million people globally. Besides children, women of reproductive age and pregnant women are the most susceptible.

Iodine is an element needed by the body for the production of thyroid hormone. Since the body does not make iodine, it has to become a part of the diet. A deficiency remains a constant challenge to public health in developing countries. Estimates are that about 1 billion people worldwide are at risk of this deficiency with goiter being the predominant health concern. Goiter or hypothyroidism occurs in regions of the world where the content of iodine in food and water is low. About 10 percent of the world's population is at risk because they live in high altitude regions like the Alps, the Andes, and the Himalayas with a water supply low in iodine.

In areas where goiter is endemic, the condition manifests clinically as a diffuse enlargement of the thyroid gland because the iodine deficiency is linked to a marked decrease in the thyroid hormone and a subsequent compensatory increase in thyroid-stimulating hormone which in turn is responsible for the enlargement of the thyroid. In developed countries where the uses of iodized salt and diets that contain iodine have been in vogue for years, the condition is hardly ever diagnosed. Iodine deficiency in developing countries could also have an association to PEM, causing decreased thyroid function. Additionally, the deficiency is important in women who are pregnant or nursing babies, causing miscarriages and stillbirth. There is also strong anecdotal evidence that some diets in tropical countries of Africa where cassava, which is considered a goitrogenic substance, and widely used as a staple, contributes to the development of goiters.

Common sources of dietary iodine are: Cheese, cow's milk, eggs, shellfish, soy milk, cheese, yogurt, breads, soy sauce, and iodized table salt.

Implications for Developed and Developing Countries

Pockets of hunger and malnutrition exist in developed countries, but from a public health perspective is comparatively non-threatening, since governments of those affected have made efforts to address the subject by different forms of intervention. In the United States, considered the wealthiest country in the world, the irony is exemplified by the fact that millions of Americans live in households with serious food problems relating to under-nutrition. It is obvious that this condition is not limited to the United States, but to varying degrees in just about all industrialized countries. The burden of hunger and malnutrition, however, is seen predominantly in the resource-poor and developing countries of the world, mostly located in the tropical belt.

It is important to recognize that the less developed countries of the globe have historically been concerned and economically challenged by the control of infectious diseases and the concomitant devastating impact this group of diseases has had on the different countries in Africa, Asia, Latin America, and the Caribbean. This compelling problem associated with the resources needed for the prevention and control of infectious diseases, typified by HIV/AIDS, tuberculosis, and malaria in the last three decades, has mostly ignored the proper recognition of hunger and malnutrition, and the broad consequences of these conditions on developing countries. The growing pertinence of chronic disease prevention and control also serves to overwhelm decision makers in these predominantly poor countries, begging the logical question, where does any country begin to maximize and optimize the necessary initiatives to promote sustainable public health in countries stressed by poverty, poor sanitation and hygiene, limited governance and infrastructure, blatant inequity, sparse resources, high unemployment, and a limited job market. These conditions are cumulative and have become so ingrained in the lives of the inhabitants of poor countries that hope becomes truly challenged.

The experience of most is that so little truly changes that expectations are seldom a part of future dreams. Since the future is nothing but a dark cloud, hopelessness becomes the norm, and life and living takes on that cycle of nothingness and the destroyer of dreams for a better tomorrow. Meals are routinely missed, simply because the forces of poverty are so pervasive that in many homes one meal a day could be a luxury. Equally disturbing is the fact that when meals do become a reality, they mostly lack the needed nutrients to provide energy, thus contributing to the endless cycle of hunger and malnutrition.

The sad reality is that regardless of the extent of the health-disease related problem, the developing countries due to poor resources to respond and the widespread poverty remains a dilemma for national governments, international governments like the World Health Organization and the Food and Agriculture Organization, NGOs, and foundations. The problems of hunger and malnutrition only add to the tremendous burden that has to be faced. The historical record provides only guarded optimism, because the challenges are so insurmountable in some of the poorest countries.

Protein-energy malnutrition (PEM) continues to be the epicenter of hunger and malnutrition discussions at the global level. Infants and young children are the most affected by PEM's impairment of growth and development, because they belong to the age group with high energy and protein demands. Additionally, hunger and malnutrition amplifies the influence of just about every disease, especially infectious diseases like measles and malaria, contributing to about 160 days of illness in young children. The complex nature of the challenge is heightened by the fact that children in developing countries are born into an environment where risk factors persist, contributing to a continuity of problems that are difficult to marginalize or prevent.

A World Health Organization report on PEM indicated that the condition affects about 25 percent of children worldwide with concomitant high levels of underweight and stunting, especially in Asia and Africa. The report further characterizes the nature of the deficiency by highlighting the correlation of PEM in the fetus during pregnancy or pre-birth to mothers who are malnourished. The major risk is borne by the fetus and could be a mixture of prematurity and low birth weight, plus the increased incidence of children coming into the world too early or too small being hampered by long-term health problems that include respiratory distress, poor immunity, and a higher than expected death rate. This affirms the problem that many children in developing countries start life at a distinct disadvantage, often with little hope of catching up. This continues to defy the best efforts of public health nutritionists in the resource-poor countries of the world.

People who are malnourished and hungry swim in a sea of hopeless hope and have a difficult time relating to lofty objectives in declarations ensuring shelter, food, and medical care to those in need. While just about all goals addressing the needs of the hungry and malnourished are well-intentioned and uplifting, the affected are really only concerned about whether or not there is a chance that they can eat something today to ward off the pains and ravages of hunger. It should be a lesson-learnt that Mother Teresa never had time to posture or declare goals and indulge in defined objectives or declarations about dealing with the poor and hungry. She and those around her spent their time more satisfying – they went out and they fed, and they ministered, and they sheltered, and they comforted. No time for lofty words other than love for those in need to assure some relief and enhance dignity. And, they did what they did with very limited resources!

There are compelling findings that there have been some improvements in the reduction of the hunger – malnutrition complex in some developing countries, but in some regions of the world the problem has actually worsened, particularly in countries of sub-Saharan Africa, and south Asia, and the depressing statistic that nearly one-sixth of all people on earth suffer from chronic hunger in the less developed countries. Many countries are plagued by emergencies from varying causes and are often in need of an immediate supply and distribution of food to ward off famine and starvation.

Discussion

The subject of hunger and malnutrition has been debated for centuries and remains a complex and challenging subject at the dawn of the 21st century. This continuum begs the obvious question, what policies or programs are needed from a global perspective to contribute to measurable improvements and change? The broad public health consequences of hunger and malnutrition in developing countries (and some developed countries) continue to mock our past and current corrective attempts. Poverty remains the principal cause of hunger and malnutrition, and it would be senseless to think that any progress can be made without an assault on poverty – associated with lack of basic resources, extreme inequity in income distribution within countries and globally, including the depressing reality that one-sixth or more of all inhabitants on earth live on $1 or less a day. Cumulatively, these socio-economic conditions and circumstances contribute to the suffering of chronic hunger and malnutrition in the resource-burdened countries, and the concomitant prevalence of widespread deficiency diseases like PEM in children and adults.

These conditions continue to exist in a world that produces enough food for everyone. Hunger and malnutrition also becomes a sword with many edges because the victims lose the ability to work efficiently and be involved in economic pursuits to assist them escape the yoke of poverty, and, optimistically, an improved standard of living. The Food and Agriculture Organization (FAO) estimates that global agriculture produces 17 percent more calories today on a per capita basis than it did three decades ago, despite a 70

165

percent increase in population. While, we are logically fixated with the concerns about protein and calories, there is the widespread problem of vitamin and mineral deficiencies affecting one third of all people living in developing countries, contributing to serious health outcomes as a result, and devoid of a clear direction or a collective workable solution to the plight of people in developing countries and the nutritional diseases that affect them.

Hilde Frafjord Johnson, Norway's former Minister of International Development and Human Rights, in one of her passionate advocacy addresses on the necessity to alleviate hunger and malnutrition amplified the serious challenges and dilemma the global public health community faces in the effort. She described the challenge as one of the most daunting of the 21st century and postured that we simply cannot refuse to become involved in the fight against poverty, hunger, and malnutrition. While logically recognizing that there are no simple solutions or quick fixes to the complexity, she proposed that national policies must give top priority to the interests of poor and starving people, and that governments must take the lead responsibility for action in their own countries. She theorized further that the overall objectives should go beyond just feeding people. The long term success will depend on the initiation of sustainable programs and systems that would help people to feed themselves. This approach would possess the "traction" needed for agricultural growth, development, and increased productivity within poor countries, will open up opportunities for jobs, and supplement the global objectives to eliminate hunger and malnutrition.

Irony adds perspective to the topic. In the developed countries, it is not unusual for increased morbidity and mortality due to conditions associated with excessive food intake, like obesity, diabetes, cardiovascular, and other like conditions, while over a billion people in the developing world go to bed hungry every night, many suffering from nutritional deficits that threaten health and well-being. I cannot help but be reminded of the famous Irish playwright and social critic, George Bernard Shaw, who postured on depressed living conditions in the early 20th century with alarm: "Do not waste your time on social conditions. What is the matter with the poor is poverty."

Conclusion

Regardless of the continuing assessments over the decades, and the interpretations of the findings, one constant factor remains a distinct challenge in every consideration of global hunger and malnutrition, and it is poverty. There is clear evidence that a nutritional divide between the rich and the poor countries, and within countries, continues to exist in spite of all forms of programs to correct the divide that have been in place for the last three or more decades. The picture in developing countries, in general, is one of under-nutrition – low birth weight in newborns, malnutrition and stunting among children, severely poorly nourished adults, widespread vitamin and mineral deficiencies, pandemic anemia, lack of access to clean water, the paucity of purchasing power for food, and marked inequity. The comparatives between the developed rich countries and the resource poor countries can be better understood in the context of diseases of affluence and diseases of poverty. The principal cause of hunger and malnutrition remains poverty. The long-term charge that we continue to face is whether we can ever truly bridge the gap between the haves and the have-nots of the world that will one day make life more worthwhile and hopeful for the latter. Can some of the excesses of the rich countries ever be channeled to serve the needs of the populations in poor countries to help overcome the plight of the hungry and malnourished? Is it being overly optimistic to state that hunger and malnutrition is unnecessary and should be deemed intolerable in the 21st century in a world where millions still die annually of hunger and malnutrition! Can we truly become a part of a concerted partnership, unified and committed, that will serve all people in a manner to help them enjoy their full potential for a better life? We must contribute to change to alleviate, and, hopefully, one day, eliminate hunger and malnutrition, and the time is now! A final thought – long term alleviation of world hunger and malnutrition is rooted in the marginalization and control of poverty because world hunger is the most classical symptom of poverty. Do we as a global community have the will, or do those who live with hope die of hunger?

"To me, a world without poverty means a world in which every person can take care of his or her basic life needs. In such a world, nobody will die of hunger or suffer from malnutrition. This is a goal world leaders have been calling for, for decades, but they have never set out any way of achieving it...

"Each day, some 35,000 children around the world die from hunger-related diseases. In a poverty-free world, no children would die of such causes. All people would have access to education and healthcare services because they would be able to afford them.....finally, a poverty-free world would be economically much stronger and far more stable than the world is today."
Muhammad Yunus, founder of the Grameen Bank

"Access to food and other resources is not a matter of availability, but rather of ability to pay. Put bluntly, those with the most money command the most resources, while those with little or no money go hungry. This inevitably leads to a situation whereby some sections of humanity arguably have too much and other sections little or nothing. Indeed, globally the richest 20 percent of humanity controls around 85 percent of all wealth, whilst the poorest 20 percent control only 1.5 percent."
Ross Copeland, The Politics of Hunger, September 2000

Don A. Franco

Chapter 8

Sustainable Food Production for Improving Health in Developing Countries

Introduction

The challenging and continuing long-standing problems of the developing countries, exemplified by poverty, and the concomitant pathologies of hunger, malnutrition, and disease, including the inefficiencies often caused by poor governance and inequity dictate that even though some debatable reports have implied a decrease in the number of hungry and malnourished in some countries, there is really very little to celebrate overall from a global perspective. Global assessments show that an increase and sustainable effort will be required for decades if there is going to be any progress or likely success of providing adequate food security to the rising populations of the resource-poor countries where hunger and malnutrition remains a continuing and compelling problem. Sustainable food production has to become the logical prioritized policy option in developing countries if there is any hope to correct this inequity. The long-term benefits of food production have been expounded as mantras for years, but still remain in the domain of the unaccomplished in so many countries that could benefit from the objectives and outcomes of sustainable food production. This goal would require maximizing and optimizing in applicable regions of developing countries the enormous potential that agricultural diversity offers through embracing and promoting new technologies like genetic advances to increase crop and livestock yields, including the other broad acceptance and utilization of biotechnology in general to improve other aspects of food production that would ensure sufficient food availability for the future.

For most marginal societies globally, agricultural improvements and other planned strategic policies involving the farming community could be the stimulus needed, not only for producing food, but to help create new livelihoods and meaningful careers in agriculture, and energize economic growth in the process. The success of these forces working in tandem could contribute to needed long-term socio-economic benefits, some job opportunities, rural development and some degree of empowerment, and an improvement in the well-being of communities through collaborative endeavors. The health status of the predominantly poor in the agricultural sector of developing countries would be beneficiaries if sustained food production is a success, because food remains in many poor countries, the single most challenging expenditure for many families. And, health could never be truly realized without a reliable and constant safe food supply.

Defining the Objectives of Food Production

Food remains essential to human existence and vital for life. In fact, food and nutrition combined are important components of

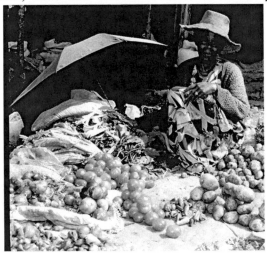

global public health and preventive medicine. Humans, by their very nature, throughout their lifespan, need a food source to supply energy, and the essential nutrients for life, growth, and reproduction. While examining the benefits of sustainable food production contextual

170

to improving health in developing countries, the broad issue of food policy/politics, globalization of agriculture, world trade and economics must also be brought into focus because of the significant implications for health, especially with pertinence to the developing countries and their individualized public health initiatives. The maintenance of natural resources and the environment in general are absolute requirements for the progress and success of sustainable production of food. This will remain a distinct challenge in many resource-poor countries, and often requires technical and economic support from donor countries and international foundations, like the Bill and Melinda Gates Foundation, to proceed with planned strategies to accomplish those objectives. In fact, this form of collaboration offers the greatest benefits for the growth and development of agriculture and food security in most developing countries where agriculture is cherished by traditions and customs, especially in Africa and Asia.

The current bountiful food supply has been influenced mainly by the rapid modernization of agriculture that has taken place in the developed countries during the past sixty years or so. The developing countries need to pursue the same direction with intensity, because the increased food production was not limited to industrialized countries. The "green revolution," particularly in rice production/technology/ and research that resulted in substantial increased yields took place in developing countries in the 1960s, and contributed to the tremendous growth in the world's food inventory. Global food supplies today are a direct reflection of the successful innovations in food production over the years, being able to meet the nutritional requirements of the world, if food was distributed based on needs. The developing countries played a meaningful role in the food production progression, and must continue to do so by objectifying this activity as a committed long-term mission of economic development and self-sufficiency.

Future projections tend to be optimistic, even in a world of widespread uncertainty, indicating that per capita food supplies will continue in an upward spiral over the next two decades. These encouraging forecasts revolve around the continuous technological innovations taking place in mostly developed countries. Fortunately, these improvements have also emerged and spread in many developing countries. In the process, these successes have enhanced agricultural development and growth in the food production chain. In spite of these forward-looking progressive trends, global sustainable food production will depend on whether or not food productivity, particularly in resource-poor countries, can meet long-term demands without a negative impact on the environment and the agricultural resources of many emerging countries. This could influence whether populations in the less developed countries would have access to enough food to pursue a healthy and productive life. These obvious concerns remain challenging as we consider the most logical path to sustainable food production to curtail hunger and malnutrition and ensure health and socio-economic national development.

The solution to the global crisis of hunger, disease, and the promotion of health must look beyond some of the traditional correctives like sending emergency food aid to countries in acute need. While this type of assistance is both valuable and moral, and always welcome, especially in affected countries ravaged by famine and other dire needs like acute starvation and the care of refugees and the blight of drought, the long-term alternative has to be self-sufficient food production to eliminate dependency. As a point of interest, in spite of claims of successful United Nations' policies to increase food production and combat hunger, the number of hungry people worldwide continues to increase with 80 percent of those affected living in rural areas with access to agricultural land for raising crops and livestock. Why is this combination of natural resources (the availability of land) and human resources, not fully exploited as a policy consideration by developing countries to enhance the goal of sustainable food production? This is puzzling and should change. The combined resources of land and people, structured as a corrective intervention, properly financed and supported by national governments, donor countries, and NGOs, could be beneficial in ways that would have a positive and lasting impact at both a local and national level. This form of innovative self-sufficiency is what developing countries need for continued forward-momentum to economic dependence. Agriculture is a big part of the road to true economic independence, and while improving human health has never been an explicit objective of agriculture in most developing countries, the association of agriculture, nutrition, and health is so obvious that it must become ingrained in global health policy.

Some of these suggested policies for change will depend on national governments investment in agricultural initiatives, especially sustainable food production, as priorities in the long-term development strategies of countries. There is no room for continued rhetoric. Nothing short of purposeful commitment and well-structured programs with both short-term and long-term objectives will succeed. These goals must be supplemented by research, something sadly deficient in developing countries due to limited financial resources, and trained personnel. Research should be applied to examine the best crop varieties, and the introduction of livestock and poultry breeds that would readily adapt to the "challenged" environments characterized by poor and limited land and water resources of most of the developing countries. Government policies must heighten the necessary incentives that would help poor, but dedicated farmers, move beyond the limits of mere subsistence. These policies have been discussed from different aspects for decades and remain a sad reminder and a poor commentary that we have to continually repeat them. We must move beyond talking and start doing, otherwise, we would not contribute to the changes needed to make agriculture, food production, and human health a successful link.

Governments have the responsibility to serve as active catalysts to expedite agricultural policies. Otherwise, little progress will be realized in achieving the objectives of a sustainable food system to assist the alleviation of hunger and malnutrition, and the improvement of health. The collaboration and cooperation of donor countries and organizations will be needed, because resource-poor countries cannot do it without the assistance to build the infrastructure it will take to achieve sustainability. But, the blind dictates of government without active re-enforcement and promotion will only result in failure. Additionally, the farming community must respond with vision and commitment to ensure success. The challenges are too complex and loaded for either the government or any form of individualism to proceed alone.

Livestock Development

The standard of living continues to improve, albeit slowly, in many developing countries, contributing to a sense of optimism for the future. In some countries, the progress is demonstrably more rapid and recognizable, while in others, there is no evidence of improvement, and in some cases there is a regression, as seen in mostly sectors of sub-Saharan Africa. The general trend in countries that show progress is a diversification of diets to include varieties of meat, eggs, and dairy products. This progression will doubtless continue as incomes rise and people migrate to the cities for jobs and opportunities for advancement throughout many developing countries, necessitating an increased demand for foods of animal origin. This emerging trend, if properly structured and managed by government could be an invaluable resource for income growth, and provide opportunities for rural communities where livestock and poultry is raised to at least examine the prospects of climbing the economic ladder through these pursuits..

This transitional opportunity, however, if not properly controlled could stress the environmental capability of many countries and exacerbate public health problems. This can be avoided if governments and the livestock/poultry industry can work collaboratively and plan objectively with long-term strategies to satisfy market demands, while enjoying the benefits of improving the overall nutritional status of the country, and directly and indirectly the economic growth of the livestock sector and the rural communities.

For centuries, the domestication of animals has contributed to being a source of food, farm power, and transportation in many developing countries. The continuing pressing demand for foods of animal origin, while a progressive trend from an agricultural and nutritional perspective, has the capability to impact negatively the many resources used in livestock production. One deficit continues to be an increase in the number of animals, rather than planned improvements in husbandry, genetics, and animal nutrition that will enhance carcass weight gains, and an overall betterment in the type of animals (or poultry) produced for food. There are major exceptions to this generalization in many parts of the developing world where successful models paralleling the developed countries are taking place in livestock development. Nonetheless, the trend to larger concentrations of animals continues unabated and has caused the clearing of forests in many regions, and a resultant degradation of the land for grazing in many areas, contributing to serious long-term environmental challenges.

Another serious challenge in many developing countries has been the need, based on economic commonsense, to move livestock closer to the urban markets to limit the cost of transportation, and improve market accessibility. This new approach, even though it creates both environmental and public health challenges, obviates the use and influence of livestock dealers, transporters, and other third party interventionists that minimize the profitability of farmers. In many developing countries with a weak regulatory framework for public health and environmental protection, the increased population of animals in overly crowded urban centers has led to an increase in the incidence of diseases transmitted from animals to man (zoonoses). These diseases can only be prevented and controlled through proper surveillance and a rigorous enforcement of health regulations, mostly lacking in resource-poor countries.

The outbreaks of different strains of the avian influenza virus, and the Nipah virus in pigs in parts of Asia, with concurrent deaths to both poultry and swine handlers in affected countries, are examples of the health related concerns that government planners are confronted with in both the animal health and public health sectors. In essence, the developing countries, in their quest to establish programs for sustainable food production to address the needs of the populations served, have to spend more resources assessing the threats of animal diseases in relation to human health, and establish extension-type educational programs to assist both producers and consumers from being victims because of the occupational association to livestock and poultry.

The abuse of pesticides and the indiscriminate use of antibiotics, both as growth promoters and therapeutically, and the poor regulatory infrastructure to ascertain compliance is cause for concern. Granted, the objective is self-sufficient food production for the developing countries, but that becomes farcical if the food is not safe. There is, therefore, an absolute necessity for developing countries to improve and modernize their food inspection capabilities to conform to the fundamentals of hazard analysis and critical control points (HACCP) to assure a safe food supply. The HACCP concept can be instituted as a country's operational model with technical and professional support from developed countries, international organizations, and the global academic community. It is a logical and proven system to promote a safe food supply. The recognition and realization of HACCP as a country's food production resource would introduce a sequential system of preventive controls that will meet many of the requirements of importing countries, thus enhancing the potential for exports, the generation of revenue, and improvement of the domestic economy through job creation.

Foods of Animal Origin

There are close to seven billion people living on Earth today, about eighty percent living in the developing countries. In every culture, good health has been an objective of government policies, and, historically, countries throughout the world have established various rules, rites, and practices to protect health. The estimated current annual population growth worldwide is about 90 million, most of this taking place in developing countries. Human beings, therefore, especially those in resource-poor regions of the globe, remain the focused epicenter for sustainable health, and hope for a productive life. This goal can be achieved by the use of foods of animal origin as sources of nutrients in human diets. This is a logical consideration because nutrition is an important determinant of maintaining health, and protein calorie deficits remain a compelling challenge throughout most, if not all, developing countries.

Nutritional challenges persist throughout the developing world because the diets of most are made up of starchy staples, lacking in protein. The supplementation of diets to include milk, meat, and eggs will help provide the protein needed, calcium, and other minerals and vitamins, and nutrients, so lacking in poor countries. Thus, the objectives to make livestock development and foods of animal origin central to planned sustainable agricultural development are based on the nutritional benefits. For example, a small poultry enterprise could be easily phased into the backyard of many rural dwellings at comparatively low cost as a start-up investment with growth potential if properly managed. The same applies, to a degree, to the raising of small ruminants, like sheep and goats. Goat milk can serve as a nutritional resource, and a source of meat when applicable.

All developing countries need programs that will invest in improving both population health and the environment. A sustainable food production system will meet those objectives. There are, however, serious deterrents to establishing a long-term and successful livestock development program in most countries, without the commitment and collaboration of government, the private sector, assessment of needs, strategic planning, and in many instances, the financing and involvement of external sources of support. A constant in developing countries continues to be the contrasts between success and failure, hopes and reality, what is and what can be! Unfortunately, while many rural inhabitants of developing countries have a genuine and traditional affinity to agriculture, including livestock farming, the cost to establish such enterprises is often prohibitive – the procurement of foundation stock, the cost of land, the cost of equipment and construction of buildings are exorbitant and beyond the means of most governments and the private sector. As a result, progressive livestock farming endeavors are mostly initiatives of big corporations, often with external sources of financial funding. This has the tendency to leave the local farming community at the periphery of sustainable livestock development, and socio-economic growth. This marginal role limits poor farmers to what I have described earlier as hopes and reality, limiting their goals to small poultry production, the rearing of goats, and in some instances, a few cattle and pigs.

The nutritional deficits of developing countries, while extremely challenging, are often complicated and compounded by the inadequacies of housing, education, and income inequity. Food production is sufficient and adequate in some countries to meet the basic energy requirements of the population, but the foods are beyond the reach of most because of poverty, particularly the protein-rich foods of animal origin that are more expensive, bordering on prohibitive. This tends to perpetuate the poverty cycle and the resulting consequences of just about everything that poverty touches – from the availability of food at affordable prices, hunger and malnutrition, disease prevalence, social and economic inequality, and even that universal hope of equal justice.

Cumulatively, poverty plus nutritional deficiencies, contribute to the diminished immune competence of the hungry and malnourished, and a greater susceptibility to infectious diseases, the main cause of death in young children in developing countries, and a constant complication of morbidity in adults. These conditions remain a daily affront to public health programs in all developing countries. The situation is very acute in sub-Saharan Africa and some Asian countries where per capita incomes are some of the lowest in the world. The broad variables that exist among the developing countries necessitate that correctives must be based on the individual circumstances, conditions, and needs of countries.

Don A. Franco

Vegetable Production as a Sustainable Resource

While there is a tendency to heighten the attributes of livestock agriculture and foods of animal origin as progressive resources for developing countries, vegetable production has in many regions the potential to be a diversified supplemental source of food. The practice of low-input sustainable production of vegetables could in many countries serve as a profit center to small farming operations, and in the process help improve the standard of living and the overall quality of life in rural communities. The irony in many poor countries is that it is easier to obtain imported cereals like wheat than some of the traditional staples like cassava, plantains, and sweet potatoes. The growing of vegetables could also have environmental benefits by helping to reduce soil loss from water and wind erosion which is a serious challenge in most tropical regions of the globe – the epicenter of the developing countries.

A vegetable agenda is in most cases also a natural fit for many regions of the world like Africa and Asia where indigenous vegetables grow easily, and at limited to no cost, and can be handled within families without disruption of the daily routine. These forces, successfully implemented, can play a significant role in the alleviation of poverty, hunger and malnutrition in developing countries through promoting vegetable production as a programmed priority, including the application of technological advancements of genetic varieties with improved disease resistance and stress tolerance, and the integration of crop, fertility, and pest control management – hazards of the climate in developing countries. This approach could help millions of farmers in the poor countries raise vegetable crops using improved varieties of seed and technologies not only for healthy diets, but to generate stronger economies that would assist national governments in their food production initiatives.

The planting and harvesting of crops like avocados, tomatoes, eggplants, cucumbers, cassava, sweet potatoes, and other like produce that fits into small scale farming, could go a long way into the improvement of agricultural productivity, potential profitability, a reduction in environmental degradation, and, hopefully, a creation of jobs, and the improved nutrition of the community/population and food security through the sustained diversification of high-value vegetables. The introduction of these crops into the commodity chain can provide a high return on investment, but will require knowledge, effective use of emerging technology, organization, and commitment to overcome some of the inherent risks like the losses entailed in both quality and quantity due to inadequate post-harvest storage, and the paucity of processing facilities.

Since people in developing countries, with few exceptions, spend about 50 to 80 percent of their disposable income on food, the option for sustainable vegetable production must be considered a logical objective to increase both the short and long-term income of small farmers, while contributing to the planned efforts for sustainable production. There is the additional encouraging benefit of the quick return to the investment of time and other resources needed to succeed, and the ultimate – the enhanced availability of food and micronutrients through vegetable consumption to alleviate hunger and malnutrition, and the likelihood of health promotion in the process.

Marine Fisheries and Aquaculture as Sources of Protein

There has been growing evidence in the last three decades that the world's major fisheries are in crisis, due mainly to the unnecessary overexploitation and depletion of sources of the fish supply. The wanton disregard of fish companies and commercial fishermen in many regions of the world for failure to properly manage the natural oceanic fish resources at sustainable levels has resulted in a threatening decrease in the existing supply. The projections for the future are not encouraging unless a concerted effort is made by all countries, especially the developing ones, to monitor through enforced regulations an effective management system, through compliance with guidelines which will assure the

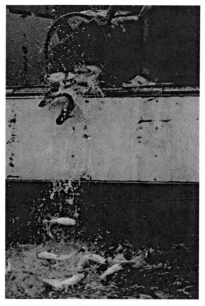

maintenance of a sustainable supply of finfish and shellfish. The realization and acceptance that the oceans are both open access and a haven for all to use as a resource for food, does not negate the responsibility and accountability of national governments and the international community from pursuing programs for sensible restraint and the prevention of abuses. Responsible action will put an end to the current excesses that are taking place in the oceanic fishing industry, and, if successful, could in time bring the fish supply into acceptable sustainable levels. According to FAO, only 6% of all marine fisheries are under-exploited, 20% moderately exploited, 50% fully exploited, 15% over-fished, 6% depleted, and 2% recovering, preventing "an efficient, equitable and transparent management of fishing capacity."

The existing circumstances of many developing countries bordering oceans and burdened by poverty and scarcity of protein sources, limiting fishermen and the oceans to recover will not be easy. The fishing industry is often the only economic outlet and means of livelihood for people in these communities. Without meaningful alternatives, the future will not be bright or encouraging for the oceans or the fish, and the people who are dependent on both.

In most developing countries with access to oceans, the governments lack the capability, resources, infrastructure, or other reasonable options to modify the conditions and circumstances that would improve the plight of coastal dwellers. Irony often comes with an ill-affordable price. While fish contains the protein with the necessary essential amino acids required by the body for growth and maintenance, and could contribute to a sustainable food and economic resource for developing countries, the current problems caused by overfishing could threaten both health and the economy in regions that could least afford that impact.

Aquaculture is nothing more than aqua-farming under controlled conditions. It has been practiced by many ancient societies like China for millennia. The overexploitation and resulting stagnation of the oceans' fish species have provided limitless opportunities for the commercial domestication of many marine species, contributing to the accelerated growth of global aquaculture to approximately 31 percent of the world's total production. This growth and expansion of the industry is nothing short of phenomenal, exceeding 10 percent per year for most species. China provides additional perspective of what is taking place. The country's foresight to make aquaculture an investment priority has paid-off beyond expectations. China now produces 70 percent of the world's farmed fish, a lot of which is exported, serving as a tremendous source of revenue that is recycled back into research and future growth and development of the industry.

Aquaculture has the additional potential of helping the sustainable production of fish as a strong economic base, especially in countries of Southeast Asia and Latin America, where aquaculture has become a part of the forward-looking food production agenda of many countries. This assists as an added boost to job creation, providing opportunities for an improved standard of living, while producing a rich protein food for consumption at home, and entrance into the export markets if applicable of a product that is in great demand. Reverting to China as an example – the thought that one country through will and strategic planning could produce 70 percent of a commodity globally should give other countries an insight of what is possible and sufficient reason for emulation.

In sectors of the world, particularly the rice-growing regions of Asian countries, there are research findings that encourage the promotion and integration of fish production to the growing of rice.

While this emerging field of rice-fish culture is limited globally, this type of production could be applicable in areas where rice is an economically important crop, and the introduction of fish could be an economic and management consideration for rice farmers, providing both additional food and income. In its simplest form this option can be readily practiced by small rice farmers, - "wild" fish enter the rice paddies during flooding of the fields and are "captured" during the end of the rice growing season during harvesting. This could assist the small farmers in the rural regions, predominantly poor and with limited resources, as a cottage industry initially, but has the potential for long-term commercialization during the rice growing and harvesting periods.

Discussion

The complex subject of sustainable food production globally, considered contextual to marginalizing poverty and improving health, remains a mocking affront to the ingenuity of the world's public health leadership. The diversity of the topics is defiant, and it is also impossible to delve into specific aspects when the planet is considered a unit for the discussion. No two countries are truly similar, but efforts were made to identify and magnify the broad potential of sustainable food production, the nutritive value of animal and fish proteins and vegetables as significant dietary attributes of populations in developing countries where hunger, malnutrition, and disease prevalence takes a heavy toll on the inhabitants. There is strong evidence that with proper strategic planning, prioritizing, and management, improvements in the food production cycle in many developing countries could influence positive changes in agricultural practices, improved nutrition, economic growth, and a likely better standard of living for some communities, ultimately improving health and well-being as the desired outcomes.

Sustainability of food production has distinct advantages as an agricultural imperative, and is relevant to protecting the future of growth and development in developing countries. While the benefits are beyond debate, challenging frustrations and problems exist – how does one logically explain and convince people living on one dollar or less a day to be conscious of the overexploitation of oceanic fishing? The same question applies to the raising of livestock and crops when the pressing needs for food to merely survive are so acute. The last consideration of the very poor in so many of the affected countries hoping for sustained food production is the attributes and potential of the concept. Their hope is often very simple and nothing more than eating today and going to bed after a meal, and avoiding the pangs of hunger, hopelessness and nothingness!

There is good reason for the continued highlighting of the distress of the resource-poor countries and the problems of the people living in these regions of the world. But, hunger is more ubiquitous than recognized. In the United States, one of the richest countries of the globe, if not the richest, adds perspective to the subject. Unknown to many is that about 35 million Americans (a little over 10 percent of the population) go to bed hungry every night. While this comparative pales to the evidential circumstances of people in developing countries, it serves as a terrible reminder that hunger, in its varying forms, approximates a universal challenge, in need of a focused corrective global agenda, recognizing that we are far from any hope of a sustainable global food production system. We do have, nonetheless, a mix of systems that are poorly linked, mostly incompatible, and very few truly sustainable.

An analysis by Pinstrup-Anderson of the challenges of a sustainable food system provides an excellent description and insight of the situation globally: "Sustainability must be measured in terms of well-being of current as well as future generations. A sustainable food system must make a sufficient quantity of safe and healthy food available to all the people it is supposed to serve, in a manner that maintains its capacity to do so for future generations. To be global, a food system must link community and natural food systems in some identifiable and internally compatible way." The thought is to protect the future - you may be living in it!

There is obvious disparity between food production agriculture in poor and rich countries, and the differences in achieving sustainability necessitate an understanding of the unique existing challenges and constraints that countries, developed or developing, have to work with in order to program for success. The industrialized countries can readily establish and follow priorities because of their resources and operational infrastructure, while the situation in the resource-poor countries is just the opposite. Nonetheless, even though the attributes of sustained food production would be a definite improvement with long-term benefits, there is really no magic solution to end the problem of hunger and malnutrition, and the cumulative ill-health linked to these conditions in the less developed countries. It would be in the best long-term interests of each developing country to analyze and base its options for program objectives on the resources and capability (ies) to achieve sustainability in food production. There would be plenty of variables to work with to realize the progress of planned goals, but, if developing countries are truly intent to follow a policy of food sustainability that will result in a sufficient quantity of safe and healthy food for all the people they are supposed to serve, success will take time and will not be fully accomplished in some parts of the world for many years, even with draconian efforts, because of the need for the development and management of a coordinated agricultural infrastructure and the necessary improved resources to make sustainability a reality.

Hurdles should never deter the collective resolve of developing countries toward systems for sustainable food production. In spite of what will appear to be impossible challenges in the pursuit, the fact is that poor countries, with food agriculture potential, cannot afford not to embrace this policy because it remains a logical and rewarding long-term option for development and economic growth. It would parallel being irresponsible, based on the needs of the people in developing societies if affected governments did not devote the energy and time necessary to enjoy the likely outcomes of food production in a sustained manner. Sustainable food production is one of the most worthy and applicable goals needed to fight and alleviate the perils of hunger and malnutrition, poverty, and disease, while contributing to improved health of millions in the less-developed countries.

Success is dependent on governments working in unison with poor and marginal farmers to incentivize and move beyond the current farming practices that involve mere subsistence farming to progressive and sustainable programs with consideration of the best crop varieties, soil maintenance, the application of scientific methods and genetics to improve aquaculture, livestock breeding and poultry production using research and genetic traits to improve yields. This impetus must be viewed as an imperative to help developing countries overcome the uncertainties of dependency and the indignity of perpetual poverty. As customary of international government agencies/bodies, inflated objectives and well-meant impressive sounding declarations are not going to do it! We have been there for decades without measurable success. The present need reverts to very modest proposals but with potentially beneficial outcomes – bring the people in the farming communities of the developing countries and their governments together – communicate, collaborate, and plan together as a unified force by examining methods to make food production in all its dimensions sustainable. The reality is that there are many countries with limited resources and progress will be slow at best. Commonsense dictates, however, that we are going to have to do the best with what exists and make expectations based on limits with a strategy for continuous improvement. That approach has to be a part of the vista for change if improvements are going to be accomplished. Tomorrows must be viewed with hope and commitment to create change if we plan to ever bury the pervasive cycle of widespread nothingness that destroys dreams.

Conclusion

Transitions of any national program are never a simple process in any country, and attempts to introduce sustainable food production and elements of agricultural diversity could be challenging and burdensome for most developing countries that are intent to overcome the widespread prevalence of hunger, malnutrition, and disease, and improve the health of people nationally. A global and sustained food supply system, while a most worthy and noble objective, would be arduous for most developing countries, but the option not to prioritize such an objective would not be forward-looking or progressive. Developing countries, regardless of the perceived barriers or limited resources, must consider these initiatives from a realistic perspective, working within the confines of available resources, while objectifying for the existing and future needs of their countries. This should parallel a mandate. The benefits and nutritive value of proteins, the potential for vegetable agriculture, and the cultivation of grains must be considerate factors into the long-term strategic plans for sustainability.

These challenging facets can only be realized through long-term commitment, and a studied recognition of the optimal and maximal use of tight resources. Good governance, management, cooperation and collaboration must be an integral part of the long-term planning needed to achieve self-sufficiency and sustainability of food production. The advantages of environmental responsibility must play a primary role, regardless of how difficult this could be for many emerging economies. Good management of natural resources and the environment are integral and compatible with food production sustainability. Additionally, the developing countries need programs that will invest in improving people's health, and economic opportunities. This is in concert with the Universal Declaration of Human Rights that posits everyone "has the right to a standard of living adequate to maintaining the health and well-being of themselves and their family, including food, clothing, housing, healthcare, and the necessary social services." Now is neither the time for indifference or silence in a world that is drowning in need.

"One of the ways we can improve exports and expand the benefits of biotechnology is to encourage countries to develop regulatory systems based on science, not politics. Unjustified and impractical legal obstacles are stopping genetically-enhanced crops from saving millions from starvation and malnutrition."
Jose W. Fernandez
Assistant Secretary of State for Economic, Energy and Business Affairs.
October 8, 2010, Washington, D.C.

"There is no medicine against fear."
Scottish proverb

Don A. Franco

Chapter 9

The Challenges for Public Health in Developing Countries

Introduction

Poverty has historically excluded the people of the developing countries (the majority of the world's population), the opportunities to enjoy the amenities and benefits of good functional health care systems, and the contributions of their inputs in the decision-making processes that could influence, mediate, and affect their health, as practiced in most industrialized countries. The continuing objectives of developing countries to build and improve their societies and enhance the overall well-being of the people would continue to defy the best intentions of public health authorities because of the disproportionate number of inhabitants that still suffer or are prone to diseases during the prime of their productive lives. This historical disparity should be corrected to permit people in developing countries the negotiating capabilities for their voices to be included in the strategic decision-making goals and policies of public health practice that will address the broad existing inequalities and program deficiencies, and, hopefully, improve the health and welfare of affected people in the future.

The major challenges in developing countries will likely continue to be infectious and parasitic diseases as they remain the prevalent concerns, concomitant with hunger/malnutrition, high fertility, especially in the Middle East and sub-Saharan Africa, and the serious problem of chronic diseases that have burdened the public health infrastructure of all countries, especially resource-poor countries. This leaves decision-makers charged with disease prevention and control responsibilities, health promotion and maintenance, wondering about the most workable measures and

189

solutions for progress and success in an era of global uncertainty, compounded by economic stresses, and limited resources. Successful interventions will depend on how well the developing countries and their support mechanisms, donors, can build on infrastructure and governance to introduce the basics of efficient primary health care and the establishment of applicable low-cost technologies to maintain and sustain the prioritized objectives for controlling and preventing the widespread incidence of infectious and chronic diseases, and improving and sustaining the health of the people. The elements needed to succeed must consider as basics: identifying the major disease problems and the concurrent costs entailed for effective intervention; establishing a health care delivery system that promotes principles to amplify primary health care strategies; defining and promoting what governments will do to ascertain that programs have the resources needed to meet both the identified objectives and the demands of the public.

The impasse, contributing to a deterrent in developing countries, particularly the least developed and the poorest, is the lack of a public health personality and the ability to build on social capital, which requires the resources and commitment to perform proper measures and analyses of the overall health system, and best methods for effective interventions to correlate with outcome expectations based on available resources. This will have to be supplemented by epidemiological surveillance other than the traditional response used for infectious disease control, and include health education and promotion to prevent and control diseases and the heightened awareness of environmental protection as a long-term strategic plan. Cost-effectiveness must be prioritized in the funding of programs to determine and affirm that intervention strategies are worth the expenses incurred – if not, a system to examine alternatives must be introduced. Assessments of the use of drugs, vaccines, and treatments must be ongoing based on costs-benefits. In most resource-poor countries, the movement to the cities and introduction of industries, both environmental monitoring and occupational safety must be programmed to include regulatory controls to preclude hazards and risks linked to the environment and workplace. The aforementioned are valid expectations, but most health systems are limited by resources or qualified personnel to transit these types of expectations to reality. The entirety of the objectives requires gradualism, and patience, much like crossing a river by feeling the stones, bur recognizing that the river must, nonetheless, be crossed.

The broad concerns of poverty, hunger, disease must become core objectives of all public health programs in developing countries, because poverty continues to be endemic and triggers the domino impact that impedes improvements. Government policies, therefore, cannot afford to overlook the blight and pathology of poverty, and must incentivize programs that are cost-effective and properly distributed and dispensed to assist the most vulnerable and needy of society. Health constructs must also heighten sustainable programs for economic and social wellbeing as integral goals, without which, the broad public health agenda could never be truly realized.

There are pockets of evidence that many developing countries have experienced economic growth over the last two decades. The trickle-down benefits to the poor and needy appear minimal. In the poorest countries, the comparative slow to no growth has perpetuated a constant cycle of poverty, mere survival and bare subsistence, precluding the potentialities of a healthy and fulfilled life. The global public health network has increased and continues its pleas of urgency to improve the conditions of the poor and oppressed by reducing social and health inequalities and the embrace of a broader and more inclusive vision to include socio-economic dimensions of communities into the long-term public health agenda.

The Role of the Community in Public Health

Public health in developing countries, and in all countries for that matter, should promote as its core agenda, programs with forward-looking initiatives and a mission to help people achieve and maintain healthy lives, concurrent with other social and economic development activities for sustainability. Each country, regardless of its stage of development, has a responsibility to establish health systems to meet the needs of the people. This could be best accomplished through the structured framework of the community. The logic is that the community is the epicenter of everything that influences health and disease, and should become the driving element for strategic public health initiatives, collaborating with government to support health objectives, and the control and prevention of disability and disease. Both health promotion and disease prevention involve careful determinants of causal factors that are best assessed at the community level. Additionally, the community brings together people at home, school, church, work and play, providing a near perfect environment for determining the associated links to morbidity and mortality, the availability and adequacy of health care services, and the corrective interventions needed for good public health practice, and the future well-being of people.

Granted, a community is basically nothing more than people living close together in a social relationship, however, activities at the community level could spread from village to village, town to town, city to city, and have a compelling influence on how things are done or can be done within countries. There is strength and potential in unity. The hope is that with effective leadership, governance, togetherness, and commitment, the actions and interventions taken at the community level could be directed towards promoting public health initiatives, and building an infrastructure for a public health bias to serve the broad needs of people. Surveillance, risk assessments, and the other facets of epidemiology to evaluate and alleviate illnesses and diseases are directly related to the community and its ability to organize successful responses. The success of programs has a definite correlation to being intimate and knowing the health deficits of the community, the processes required to respond to challenges, and the ability to bring social forces together to sustain desired outcomes. The fact remains that within a community people often embrace common values with a sense of belonging that influences relationships and their future, including the forces that impact life, living, employment, governance, and health. The community, then, can be the resource for unifying responsibility and accountability for public health goals in developing countries. It could be an initial simple project like the promotion of childhood vaccinations at the village level that could spread to the next village or town, and ultimately the majority of the country for the greater good.

The potential of the community philosophy for public health promotion goes beyond the village or town concept. A workshop initiative held in Bangkok, Thailand, in 2003, illustrates the benefits of community action and the international impact for disease control

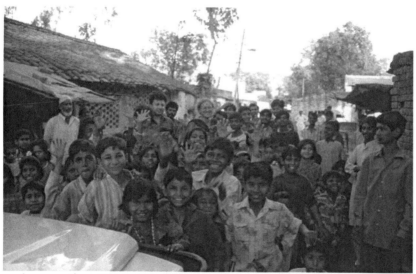

and prevention. The goal of the workshop brought African and Asian government officials together with aid workers and United Nations' personnel to examine strategies and encourage farmers from both regions how to use their occupational knowledge of agriculture to assist their communities to marginalize the transmission and consequences of HIV/AIDS, since the disease has such a threatening impact on both continents. The core objective of the workshop was to assess the role of ministries of agriculture in both Africa and Asia to assist HIV/AIDS devastated communities to pursue their farming activities, while working to assess the factors linked to a common agenda to overcome their problems, including how farmers' behaviors could expose them to the virus.

Not many people looking at the broad dimensions of community responses, and international collaboration, would consider HIV/AIDS in an agricultural context. Nonetheless, an evaluation of the possibilities of communities, in this case global in scope, South – South collaboration (Africa and Asia), puts the value of community efforts as being beyond the limits of a location, assuming that people are willing to cooperate and achieve together to conquer diseases for the sake and well-being of humanity worldwide. The potential has no barriers if we are willing as a global community to work as a unified force for the common good. The "community," therefore, could be anything that public health planners want it to be – a village, a town, a city, a country, a continent, a region, or the globe. Success really depends on political will, commitment, and infrastructure for governance by keeping the objectives realistic based on available resources.

Science-oriented Public Health for Developing Countries

In the 1960s, the world started to experience rapid social and economic improvements, at or around the same time that many countries were becoming independent, and shedding their colonial past. During this period of transition, and the emergence of new independent countries with great dreams and expectations, including the autonomy that the new status of independence offered, many of the former colonists, nonetheless, maintained an active interest in the governance, infrastructural building, and welfare of their former colonies. This was exemplified through various assistance programs with concomitant professional and technical support mechanisms with objectives for cooperative collaboration. As customary, the United Nations played an integral role as a facilitator and through its

UN Development Decade in 1961, promoted and helped to establish a philosophy for both sustainable growth and social development in this new and exciting sea of change. This was also a period of marked contrasts, because although there was evidence of encouraging economic growth and social stability, demonstrated by the obvious abundance and overall well-being of the developed countries, the compelling needs and the anguish of poverty of the predominantly poor developing countries surfaced to taunt, defy and mock the global leadership, especially in the sphere of disease prevention and control and public health initiatives.

Nonetheless, the historical ties, the commercial and cultural bonds, a sense of mutual interest, and the social interconnectedness between the colonists and their former colonies were so firmly in place that the assurances, in most cases, of a post-independence relationship were beyond doubt. The British Commonwealth serves as a perfect example. There were causes for hurt and dissent at times in past relationships with many former colonized countries and those who ruled the colonies, but the broad commonalities and bonding that have emerged over the years worked towards the current goals of mutual interest, many linked to educational endeavors for the training and development of professional staff that included public health to meet the challenges of the newly independent countries. The now independent developing countries were mostly definite beneficiaries of this association. They enjoyed the largesse of economic, educational, and technical support, and the continuous collaboration and exposure to their former colonists to the improvements of the scientific potentiality in their own countries, especially in the arena of health promotion and maintenance. Education and science-oriented public health became an important integral component of this post-independence transitional relationship. While the British Commonwealth was "isolated" for this discussion, one would be remiss not to recognize that the same existed, in varying degrees, with Spain, Portugal, Belgium, and Holland, countries that played active roles in transitional economic development and health improvement efforts in their former colonies, mostly through joint collaborations in the field of post-graduate medical education and technical support to upgrade the health infrastructure..

In nearly all the new independent countries, the challenges to meet the professional and development needs of the "locals" were compelling, especially in the field of public health. The problem was both clear and demanding – the healthcare facilities were generally inadequate to meet the needs of the populations served, particularly in the rural areas. Just about every conceivable healthcare service had to be improved if there was any hope to provide efficient basic primary care to the people. Additionally, the future staffing of public health/preventive medicine centers or clinics needed physicians and professional support personnel who were trained to promote a public health aspect/concept to care. This was sadly lacking and became a serious void that had to be corrected, and remains an affront to this day in most of the developing countries. The staffing prior to independence has traditionally been from the "mother" country, with very little strategic plans for the education of the locals to meet the future public health initiatives and preventive medicine objectives. Additionally, the historical approach has always been curative medicine. Public health/preventive medicine, therefore, has always been an afterthought, to this day, in many countries, including developed countries. So, as we seriously examine the applicability and functionality of science-oriented public health as an adjunct to overall long-term health care, it is totally apparent that developing countries have a treacherous mountain to climb. In the least developed countries, burdened by widespread and devastating poverty, and the concurrent lack of resources, the attribution of science-oriented public health to contribute to disease prevention and control becomes nothing but a dream to be realized. Disease remains the pathology of poverty, and the connectedness is so complex that developing countries hoping to benefit from the science-oriented public health concept would have to take a gradualist approach.

Science-oriented public health could play an important ancillary role in just about every aspect of health promotion and disease

Don A. Franco

control in developing countries – from the 30 percent or more who suffer from malnutrition in the least developed countries to the introduction and promotion of a vaccine for young women against the papilloma virus linked to cervical cancer, and a continuing cause of high mortality in developing countries. The success will depend on the ability of individual countries to alleviate poverty, infectious diseases with concurrent parasitism, poor governance and lack of resources, insufficient farm productivity contributing to under-nutrition, the emerging challenges of chronic diseases, and famine and civil wars where these types of conflicts prevail. Additionally, epidemiological surveillance programs to assess population health and the introduction of interventions to accommodate and respond to needs are necessary to assure positive outcomes. For science-oriented public health to be efficient and effective, many developing countries would need to create new institutions and reorganize the old ones in a manner to build capacities to conform to the concept. Gradualism and long-term commitment, despite the acute and immediate needs of the resource-poor countries, must be part of a national development strategy for each country, and could ideally help to establish science-oriented public health as an integral part of sustainability for health promotion and disease control in the future.

Disease Eradication Challenges in Developing Countries

One definition of disease eradication is "a reduction of the worldwide incidence of a disease to zero as a result of deliberate efforts, obviating the necessity for further control measures." The underlying theme of eradication is global, regardless of the targeted disease, with an outcome objective to attain "the certified total absence of human cases, the absence of a reservoir for the organism in nature, and absolute containment of any infectious source." Using smallpox as an analogy, four major factors contributed to the successful eradication of the disease:
1.   The reservoir for the virus only existed in humans.

2.   All infected persons had classical symptoms in the form of a recognizable rash, and were infectious for a relatively short period.

3.   The natural infection resulted in lifelong immunity.

4.   An effective and safe vaccine was used and was very stable in tropical environments where the majority of the cases took place and prioritized for immunization.

Smallpox was amplified for obvious reasons. The disease has become the central illuminating example of eradication of a disease. It has also become a part of the historical record of the successful accomplishments and management strategies for prevention and control of infectious diseases, and is ingrained in the annals and history of medicine. The eradication of the disease began in 1796 with Edward Jenner's experimentations that showed inoculation of the virus that caused cowpox, a cattle disease, provided immunity to smallpox in humans. The initial work of Jenner to the WHO pronouncement of eradication took 170 years, officially making smallpox the first disease for which a vaccine was successfully applied to put an end to a human scourge. This breakthrough provided optimism, inspiration, and the tonic needed to stimulate global public health and the perfect impetus to institute disease control, prevention, and possible eradication programs of other infectious diseases that threaten developing countries. The eradication of smallpox was, put mildly, euphoric for global public health. The success showed the world that determination, will, good management, and a strategic plan could break the barriers of an infectious disease.   The recognition that medical and support personnel from developing countries were active participants in the momentous accomplishment could serve as a reference for future challenges and a source of encouragement. It was a success for medical and public health globalization, the World Health Organization, and the progress for humanism and justice, because the smallpox virus infected and killed the most vulnerable and at risk people in the world, living in the least materially developed countries.

Disease eradication is global in scope. Since the burden of disease continues to be in the developing countries that lack the corrective response infrastructure to mitigate, marginalize or control diseases, without external technical and financial support of donors, the future is tenuous and has to be continuously assessed with the intent to institute improvements. This necessitates dependence and collaboration using joint ventures to advantage with international organizations like WHO, and private sector foundations like the Bill and Melinda Gates Foundation, dedicated to prevent the ravages of disease in the least developed countries, and the promotion of general well-being of underprivileged and resource-poor countries and their people. Whether or not other diseases can be eradicated like smallpox would be tested in time. A model exists to work from and some of the management principles of eradication can apply to other diseases, whether or not of a microbial nature.

Dracunculiasis ("guinea worm") has been on the "fast track" for years with encouraging results that eradication could be accomplished if the momentum and funding continues. This disease needs no vaccine intervention, is limited by geography to a few countries of the tropical regions of the world, requires only the education of people that comes relatively cheap, and is transmitted by only one reservoir, drinking water, that contains copepods (fresh water micro-crustaceans or "water fleas") which carry the infective larvae. The disease is exclusively transmitted through drinking contaminated water, and could be prevented and controlled, eliminated or eradicated by preventing people with open ulcers associated with the infection from entering ponds or wells used as a drinking water source, and the simple process of filtering drinking water by using a cloth filter to remove the copepods ("water fleas"), the carriers of the infective agent. The Carter Center of Emory University has been the lead institution in this eradication effort and deserves the recognition and credit for the tremendous success over the years in the rapid decline of the prevalence of this disease.

Can diseases like schistosomiasis ("snail fever") with an intermediate snail host, and onchocerciasis ("river blindness") transmitted by black flies and the cause of serious eye lesions and blindness, mainly in Africa, be ever eradicated? Can similar control strategies and planning used for eradicating "guinea worm" apply? Malaria continues to plague one third of the world's population, especially devastating to the children of Africa, causing excessive annual mortalities. This is linked to a depressing statistic that as many or more people die today from malaria than 30 years ago, accounting for 25-50% of all hospital admissions. Can the complex life cycle of malaria and the transmitting Anopheles mosquito ever be eliminated or eradicated? Besides being a serious global public health risk, the disease has economic and sociological implications. Is a vaccine a realistic expectation? Will WHO's Roll Back Malaria (RBM) program and similar initiatives including the outlined objectives in the current Millennium Development Goals ever result in meaningful control, elimination, or eradication of the disease? Do we truly have the collective determination and will to succeed, or do we introduce the challenges of the poverty factor and the additional vague socio-economic nuances to the lack of accomplishment? Is the elimination or eradication of tuberculosis feasible in the endemic regions of the world in the foreseeable future? Can the BCG vaccine be improved to add impetus to tuberculosis control initiatives? Disease control in developing countries continues to be difficult to define or fully understand. The high mortality associated with neonatal tetanus in children, exceeding 80%, predominantly in Africa, and

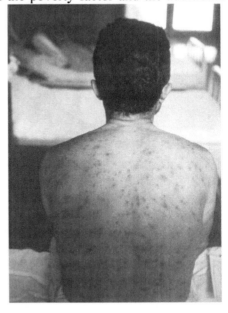

unheard of in industrialized countries, amplifies the need for collaboration and understanding of the uniqueness of diseases in the tropical world, and the mandate for global cooperation and research in tropical diseases.

Some viral preventable diseases, typified by poliomyelitis, remain ideal candidates for eradication. There are ample reasons for cautious optimism. The improved and concerted immunization programs worldwide and the conviction that eradication of polio is feasible have contributed to a dramatic reduction in the incidence of the disease globally. The costs and benefits of eradication are positive, especially in the long-term consideration of the possible cessation of polio immunization as a continuing measure, and the monetary and human resources needed for the prevention and control of the disease. Unfortunately, many of the immunization initiatives linked to eradication, like achieving 90% coverage of a susceptible population, have not been realized due to lack of political commitment and resources that are often beyond the capacity of many national governments. Successful eradication of polio in countries where the disease is endemic will depend, at a minimum, of fully supporting and sustaining programs for a minimum of 3-5 years. This has not taken place in many countries for a variety of reasons making any likely celebration of the last case of polio or the potential of eradication years away.

Measles (rubeola), the most contagious disease of mankind, is another considerate candidate for eradication. The disease is responsible for excessive deaths in developing countries due to complications of malnutrition, diarrhea, and pneumonia as concomitant risk factors. While an effective measles vaccine has been in use for over forty years, deaths associated with this disease remain a serious threat to public health in the less developed countries of the world, predominantly in Africa and Asia. The WHO estimates that measles is the leading killer of a vaccine-preventable disease of children, killing approximately one million of the forty-two million diagnosed annually. In the tropical regions of the world, with the least developed countries, children who are not vaccinated before the age of five will ultimately become infected and be part of a case fatality rate of one and five percent.

With smallpox setting the stage for new global public health initiatives and a source of inspiration to examine other options, diseases like poliomyelitis and measles are now amplified in the WHO's Expanded Program on Immunization as logical eradication targets. The decrease prevalence of polio globally in the last two decades provides cause for optimism that eradication, with a continued planned resolve, is possible. In the case of measles, one barrier remains the ease of transmissibility of the virus, and the thinking of many in the medical community of developed countries that measles is nothing more than a disease of childhood with limited morbidity and mortality consequences. Unfortunately, measles presents a different clinical picture in developing countries with high case-fatality rates that spiral to as high as thirty percent in high-risk regions in immune-compromised children.

Measles prevention and control needs a "transfusion" in the developing countries and the financial resources and technical support to move programs forward to a hope of eradication. Based on the experience of the United States and other resource-rich countries, this disease can be eradicated globally with concerted long-term prioritized programs that approximate the smallpox initiative. It should be a "Marshall Plan" type of effort – insightful and focused. The effective use of a measles vaccine has resulted in more than a ninety-nine percent reduction of cases in the United States. This success can be used as a logical basis to affirm the benefits of prevention and ultimately eradication.

We are predominantly focused globally on the eradication of diseases that can meet the parameters of the eradicating objectives, especially in the most vulnerable populations of the world – the developing countries. The preoccupation with the bacterial, viral, and parasitic diseases is logical based on the burden to health services and the morbidity and mortality. Unfortunately, the chronic diseases must be factored into the prioritization together with the deficiency diseases associated with iodine, iron, vitamin A, and folic acid as significant challenges. While eradication is not a considerate option for chronic and deficiency diseases, these diseases, nonetheless, complicate and confound the entire public health momentum and resources of developing countries.

Development Assistance for Health

There is growing enthusiasm and optimism for organized and programmed development assistance for health (DAH). The advent of the twenty-first century saw an emergence of a new source of energy and funding, exemplified to the utmost by the active, hands-on involvement of Bill and Melinda Gates, and the professional leadership and technical support staff of the Foundation they established – the Bill and Melina Gates Foundation. The early objectives of the Foundation was to work with allied groups like the World Health Organization and governments, including that of the United States, to initiate a Global Fund to fight AIDS, Tuberculosis, and Malaria, and a special commitment from the United States to a meaningful affront and financial funding for the HIV/AIDS epidemic.

It is impossible to truly analyze the impact of the Bill and Melina Gates' efforts – their active participation, political and entrepreneurial influence, defined commitment to humanity and disease control, the promotion of the concept of the dignity and equality of man, and the aspects of social justice - defy words. This Foundation is without doubt the most influencing arm for disease prevention and control objectives in the world today, providing the impetus and guidance needed to alleviate poverty and the global prevalence of disease, especially vaccine preventable diseases, and, by example, providing the "fire," leadership, financial support and optimism to assist world organizations like WHO, UNICEF, the World Bank and others to move forward together and collaborate to new heights and aspirations. The foundation also builds on hope and a positive outlook for the future of the developing countries, standing as an example for other donors and NGOs to emulate. This could have a positive influence on other sources of finance and technical support with an interest in health and economic development in resource-poor countries, providing the world's public health community cause for continued optimistic programming to improve well-being and conquer diseases in the world's most vulnerable and at risk communities.

The Gates Foundation is a positive attraction. Warren Buffett, a close family friend and one of the richest men on the planet, decided to donate billions to the programs and objectives of the foundation, providing the financial resources to make good things happen in the less developed countries. It is difficult to determine the long-term impact of the Gates-Buffet alliance, except to posture that it would add significant and important dimensions to global public health objectives. The distribution of the financial support for medical research, disease control, immunization programs, hunger and poverty alleviation, and the alliances and joint collaboration with national governments in developing countries to address population needs would be compelling!

This trend toward the uplifting of people in developing countries is spreading and "infecting" all types of celebrities from broad regions of the globe. They have become more involved in the blight of poor countries, including the glaring indignities of social injustice that so many face on a daily basis. A lot of financial support was linked to the HIV/AIDS epidemic – with understanding. But, many have recognized that the central theme of HIV/AIDS, while important, is also associated with poverty, malnutrition/hunger, and diseases that also need sustained collaborative involvement if any hopes of measured improvements are going to be realized. This is what has started to evolve at the advent of the 21st century, fueling new hope for the sustainability and funding of programs. Additionally, many donor organizations are moving towards the support of research endeavors and new technologies to assist overall development and economic growth to supplement health objectives with professional and technical support from organizations like WHO, the local health sector, and academic institutions in many developing countries. As implied earlier, while HIV/AIDS touches the emotional button easily, we also have to pursue relentlessly the devastation caused by tuberculosis, malaria, and the other neglected tropical diseases (NTDs), if we have any hope of moving forward with a new energized era of global public health to create dreams of better tomorrows for the world's underprivileged.

Africa, logically, continues to be the largest recipient of development assistance for health. This equates to an average of about 35%, followed by Latin America and the Caribbean at 14%, East and South Asia about 11%, and approximately 7% for the Middle East. The rest, about 20%, goes to different forms of program activities to other countries. These allocations of resources could and would vary over a period of time based on emergencies, war, famine, disease outbreaks, and other unanticipated factors. The percentages, however, are a fair representation and somewhat consistent of the financial distributions and support that have been extended to these different regions for the past two decades.

The major funding programs continue to prioritize the infectious diseases, and using HIV/AIDS as an example, is still woefully inadequate to counter the broad spectrum of the pathologies associated with this complex disease in developing countries, in spite of substantial progress in some countries. The development assistance for health objectified in the Millennium Development Goals (MDGs) is going to be an expensive process, and in many countries will not come close to being accomplished. The constant challenge remains bringing new technologies and upgrading the technical and professional support and resources necessary for widespread use to be able to sustain health improvement programs that would have an impact in the least developed countries. Other interventions to enhance development are good governance, optimal use of resources, building an infrastructure for effective cooperation and collaboration between the numerous sectors working on health agendas to facilitate outcomes and the involvement of the community as active participants, the training and continuing education of health personnel to increase efficiency and productivity, and a sense of accomplishment.

Discussion

While we support and advocate what disease control and prevention programs are needed to assure a progressive agenda for health promotion, especially in developing countries, success would be dependent on individual communities and the will of the people at a national level. The diverse challenges of public health dictate this to be the logical approach – cooperation and collaboration - if we have any hope of ending inequalities of the living and working conditions of the poor and destitute in the least developed countries. Remarkable improvements and successful health programs have taken place in some countries, especially in the middle income developing countries, with corrective interventions that have modified the social matrix and access to services at health clinics and hospitals. In many of the sub-Saharan African countries, the progress has been marginal to non-existent, confirming the analogy that extreme poverty causes extreme bad health. The pathology of poverty, therefore, has interesting and differential dimensions that must be studied in the context of global public health.

The community as a model for the promotion of health and the control of disease is a rational and considerate objective, since the community is the central force to bringing everything together. The community can be used as the major intervening resource for the establishment and promotion of priorities, the presentation of educational programs, strategic planning, a center for discourse, and the locus for promoting and embracing common values to amplify health. This encourages participatory debates, the assessment of options, and fosters the buy-in to programs, creating the process a unified force for the common good of people.

Science-oriented public health has become a clarion call for the progression of global public health practice and a significant impetus for activating and improving public health initiatives nationally and globally. Unfortunately, many of the developing countries, due to lack of resources, would find the concept a burden to apply, despite the apparent benefits. Many developing countries, nonetheless, much to their credit and foresight, plan to factor into their development strategies the principles of science-oriented public health to augment their disease prevention and health promotion objectives. Donors can play a contributory role through collaboration, academic cooperation, funding, and technical and professional support to make this a realized benefit.

Global disease eradication is a demanding public health objective. It is a complex and defying process, and regardless of the optimism generated during international forums, and the rapid advances in medical technology, eradication as an outcome of any disease is fraught with every conceivable barrier. Nonetheless, there are still flashing lights of hope for the future eradication of some diseases. Obvious examples are dracunculiasis ("guinea worm"), poliomyelitis, and measles – providing global public health planners compelling reasons to consider the potential for eradication. The "guinea worm" initiative is on a progressive path, fueled by encouraging results over the past two decades, heightened by the guidance, leadership, commitment, and active collaboration of the Carter Center of Emory University. Equally positive is the impressive reduction in the prevalence of polio worldwide, and the prioritization of immunizations in most developing countries, providing reason to consider eradication as having a logical chance of achievement if the current support and resolve continues. The United States can be considered as an ideal indicator and example for the potential eradication of measles through immunization. The rapid reduction of measles cases over the years to less than 1 percent incidence should support and ignite the logic for the possibility of eradication globally. A successful outcome would not come without extensive planning and good management and the proper use of resources to comply with the objectives of a high level of immunization of the at risk population.

The fact is that development assistance for health programs has presented a new and clearer path at the advent of the 21st century. A new sense of direction and opportunity has emerged, heightened by the diversity of initiatives financially supported by the Bill and Melinda Gates Foundation. While, it is obvious that this is not the only foundation committed to a change agenda for disease control and health promotion, the Gates family has shown the world how to respond to urgency and the need for immediacy in a world of dire needs. The foundation has also served as a source of "added value" to many established public health programs in developing countries to improve health and control disease in the most vulnerable populations, amplifying in the process – the dignity of every person – the humanity of humanism.

Whether or not there would ever be enough external support from private foundations and NGOs to help "turn the tide" and marginalize the negative consequences associated with the widespread prevalence of diseases in developing countries will remain unanswered for decades. The current level of consciousness and the heightened momentum that has evolved about the needed interventions to combat the ravages of poverty and disease is a source of encouragement. Granted, the global issues continue to be immense, but the Gates Foundation (and many others too numerous to individualize) have given us a path to find the road of hope and optimism. The ultimate success will be dependent on whether or not we can overcome the major challenges that global public health face by contributing through active collaboration and unity to make the world a better place for all by preventing and controlling diseases and improving health for the helpless.

Conclusion

The developed countries, in general, have already demonstrated their ability to manage the established public health infrastructures in a sustainable manner, but the developing countries, especially the least developed, will have to continue to examine new approaches and innovative interventions to improve their programs and meet defined goals of acceptability, particularly in the delivery of primary health care and the maintenance of clinics, mainly in the rural regions. A lack of adequate and sustained funding has been at the epicenter of the debate facing developing countries contextual to the success or failure of programs. There are, however, no guarantees that there would ever be sufficient resources (monetary or otherwise) to respond to the corrective needs and sustain the necessary programs to institute reforms in the future. This becomes very apparent as the challenges and complex issues that many countries face are assessed. Every continent, exemplified by Africa and Asia, has unique needs. There are reasons, nonetheless, to be cautiously optimistic and forward-looking. The new influx of funding accompanied by global consciousness that the burden of disease and health promotion is everybody's business helps the momentum to achieve reform and change. In the 21st century and beyond, health will be a global issue.

Economic growth and development, the alleviation of poverty, and the concomitant derived benefits for the potential of an improved standard of living could and would obviously contribute to progress, and some successes. This will take time and commitment and a mandate for governments' involvement and collaboration to accelerate and activate priorities for the public good. This will definitely test the mettle of most developing countries, but using the community as a model to institute change, plus the current evolution of external sources of assistance frugally and wisely, the opportunity for aspiring and achieving together becomes hopeful for so many in need that they will one day be able to enjoy better tomorrows.

"I like to see a man proud of the place in which he lives.
I like to see a man live so that his place will be proud of
him."
Abraham Lincoln

"The higher your energy level, the more efficient is your body. The more efficient your body, the better you feel and the more you will use your talent to produce outstanding results."
Anthony Robbins, 1960-

"Health, therefore, is not merely the absence of disease – it is something positive, a happy attitude toward life, and an eager acceptance of the responsibilities it entails."
Henry Sigerist, 1891-1957

Chapter 10

Is There Reason for Optimism?

The question of optimism relative to the progress and success of global health initiatives, and the quality of life, especially in developing countries, is a difficult and complex one because it entails a periscope of the past, an assessment of the present, and reflections into the future, during a period of widespread uncertainty throughout the world. In two of my previous books covering the broad realm of poverty, disease, and health, the lives and circumstances of the poor was the central theme. This book (Poverty, Hunger, Disease and Global Health) replicates many of the same concerns and challenges that continue to taunt and defy our ongoing efforts to bring meaningful change to the world's impoverished. Poverty and its interrelatedness to societies in resource-poor countries, including its relevance to hunger/malnutrition, increased incidence/prevalence of diseases, poor housing, lack of adequate educational resources, marginal and low paying jobs, and a challenged health infrastructure collectively contribute to a state of hopelessness. Additionally, the economic inequality and other elements of social injustice, directly or indirectly linked to the circumstances and consequences of poverty, make the question a challenging morass, and confounding clear answers for reasons to be optimistic.

The socio-economic and health factors and variables traditionally used to evaluate the progress of developing countries, and, within countries, defy a workable or usable model for assessments that could truly measure accomplishments or success, making the question of optimism and a reason for hope moot, and, in fact, a distinct and clear answer impossible. Attempts to make analyses at many national levels have been unreliable because of poor to non-existent data and an overabundance of anecdotes. Often,

211

the numbers used just do not correlate with anything that can be validated, even with the best technical support of organizations like WHO and the World Bank. Some countries remain so challenged in their attempts to provide basic services that analyses of functions (health or otherwise) are unreliable. Records and the process of record-keeping fail to conform to traditional standards because of the outdated systems in place. This is reality, and not meant as an indictment. It is only a symptom of the deficits of resources and the resulting limits of governance that many countries have to work with. Other countries, however, have shown impressive improvements in both the general standard of living and health. The developing countries, in general, therefore, remain a mix of trepidation and hopelessness, and optimism and hope.

The future, whether or not it provides reason for optimism and celebration, must be examined from the perspective of what we plan to do as a global health community to contribute to positive change to make life more meaningful for the poor and impoverished regardless of the severe problems and challenges that continue as thorns and barriers along the way. Many of the problems are so very basic and frustrating – in some of the least developed countries, sanitation and hygiene, health fundamentals, are worse today than decades or centuries ago. In fact, countries that are populated by more than half of the world's population, poverty continues to be the most challenging dilemma and an affront to governments' ability to maintain a sanitary and hygienic environment for people. This ongoing failure is responsible for an associated link and a domino type impact on high disease prevalence, mostly infectious, with a concurrent challenge of limited health care facilities and a public health infrastructure that is essentially in disarray and in need of restructuring.

Some countries that fall in the middle category in economic development and industrial growth have shown remarkable resiliency. This is well-exemplified by China and India with more than one third of the world's population and considered marginalized by the developed countries only a decade or two ago, have now emerged, despite pressing problems, as the epitome of hope for others to emulate. The two countries are now major players in the global economy, providing impetus for others to recognize that progress is possible dependent on determination, commitment, foresight, and will. Additionally, both countries have made concerted efforts to improve their public health infrastructure, cognizant of the severity and nature of some of the health related problems, exemplified by environmental degradation that contribute to hazards and in need of long-term strategic planning and management. In spite of the cause for celebrations linked to economic growth and development, both China and India recognize that half of the world's poor who subsist on less than $2 a day live within their borders, making optimism tentative and the need to do more imperative.

Waterborne diseases will continue to plague the countries of the developing world. A disturbing fact is that one third of the world's population living in the poorest countries has no access to safe drinking water, and in some countries in sub-Saharan Africa, potable water makes up 10 percent or less of the water supply. The public health inference is that water remains the primary vehicle of infection for cholera and other deadly infectious diseases. Unless access to clean water becomes a serious public health imperative and one day, hopefully, a reality, populations in developing countries remain at high risk and

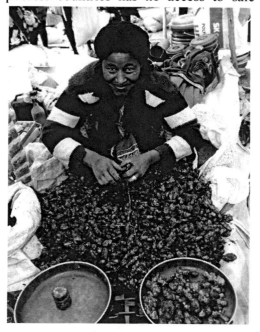

vulnerable.

Food safety assurance and the control of food-borne diseases have become a global public health imperative. Sporadic outbreaks of food-borne diseases still challenge the industrialized countries in spite of their well-organized and prevention and control infrastructure with sophisticated technical and scientific support. The developing countries, in contrast, due to limited resources, ubiquitous poor sanitation and hygiene, environmental degradation, and very marginal food inspection programs, including the lack of state of the art technology make prevention and control of food-borne diseases problematic.

Many donor countries and international organizations like the World Health Organization have worked with resource-poor countries to address the existing inadequacies through educational grants and the promotion of hazard analysis and critical control points (HACCP) principles to improve food safety. The problem is more than donor country intervention or international health organizations. The correctives necessitate the active involvement of the countries themselves to institute reform and buy-in, and, often this commitment can be without a financial burden to the affected governments. It is about responsibility, accountability, and proper program planning and prioritization.

The dilemma of infectious diseases continues to be problematic in developing countries. Many of the middle income developing countries have made impressive progress in controlling and preventing infectious diseases through immunization and other public health interventions using risk assessments, surveillance, and new technologies in diagnostics. Sadly, many countries in Africa, Asia, the Middle East, Latin America and the Caribbean need to do more to realize meaningful change – the need for clean water predominates, food safety assurances must be heightened, improved sanitation and hygiene must be a prioritized part of the public health agenda, access to health care clinics and other facilities with resources to treat those in need has to be central to national objectives including a structured implementation of vaccination programs.

HIV/AIDS and the medical and social impact of this pandemic amplify every aspect and concept of inequity and inequality. It highlights the darkness of social injustice that inhabitants of resource-poor countries have to face because of the doom of poverty, and symptomatic of the conditions in which people live. Poverty limits freedom and the epicenter of the disproportionate burden of infectious diseases. HIV/AIDS also clearly demonstrates how industrialized and developed countries can respond to a public health crisis and how woefully inadequate most of the developing countries are. The burden of the disease and the concomitant distress and suffering can only be marginalized and corrected when governments can effectively introduce programs to promote social justice as part of the national public health agenda. Can this be cause for optimism? Do we have the will?

Hunger and malnutrition will persist as a compelling challenge to the developing countries for decades and the thought of food production as a social and public health response policy must be factored into the long-term planning strategies of developing countries, WHO, UNICEF, USAID, the World Bank, NGOs and other donor agencies. The malnourished and hungry complicate efforts at health promotion because they are serious barriers to wellness. This condition exists even in a country like the United States, an epicenter of affluence and an overabundance of food, and the surprising reality that so many go to bed hungry each night – linked to the perils of poverty. Professor Sachs' theories to put an end to poverty promote optimism, but the dark clouds of reality continue to blank out many of his proposals for hope. That should not kill and bury optimism, because it is all we have left!

Chronic diseases have spiraled to the top of global health concerns. People are living longer, and the elderly have become the majority, especially in industrialized countries, and, to a degree, in many more economically advanced developing countries that now enjoy an improved standard of living. The causal association of infectious agents to chronic diseases, including some forms of cancer, should bring new energy and challenges for epidemiology, research, and assessments for prevalence. The developed countries will continue to lead the way in new findings and information through research, but ongoing collaboration with academic centers in developing countries and joint study initiatives could help developing countries address some of their problems with the control and prevention of chronic diseases. The constraint will continue to be the struggle of poor governments with lack of basic resources to respond adequately, and another logical concern, what can we do, as a global health community, to ascertain that chronic disease prevention and control initiatives will get to those in need?

Poverty remains the all inclusive generic factor that has to be alleviated before developing countries can be freed from the burden of hunger/malnutrition, disease, and the establishment of health services to meet the demands of the populations served. The developed countries now face chronic diseases as a predominant problem with heightened objectives for prevention and control programs. The developing countries will continue to be affronted by both the ravages of infectious and chronic diseases, amplified by the continuing high morbidity and mortality of HIV/AIDS. The lights do not flicker easily as we reflect on the health conditions of developing countries. Often, we are left only with our collective optimism. Logically, we will need more than that to influence the reforms and changes needed.

"Health for all" and the right to health as concepts should be promoted globally. The objectives become a myth, however, because the developing countries do not have the resources now or in the foreseeable future to make those worthy themes a reality. We must advocate the ideals but accept the existing limitations and operate within the framework of limits. We must return to the basics, because in most developing countries that would be all that we have to work with – supplying clinics and health centers with needed medicines, vaccines, and elementary diagnostic capabilities to serve the daily wants of people. We must supplement those meager basics

216

with trained support staff – nurses, doctors, laboratory technicians, midwives, to keep the community functioning while hoping to meet the minimum acceptable requirements for health care. Additionally, there is an urgent management need to organize health services in a manner not to disenfranchise those in need of health care. The many who are turned away daily because of lack of medicines, vaccines, or no professional intervention by doctors should not continue. This is not because people are indifferent to the plight of the needy, but simply because the infrastructure does not exist to maintain a semblance of efficiency. The social conditions are absent – the government is poor – the people are poor – contributing to that horrifying cycle of hopelessness to test our ingenuity.

In spite of this description of "darkness" one would have to be callously indifferent and a true pessimist not to conjure up optimism and hope, despite the pressing and depressing problems of the poor countries. The unselfish reaching out of individuals, small groups, NGOs, foundations, the religious working in church missions, schools, clinics and hospitals, the efforts of national governments and world institutions – all dedicated to helping people live better and healthier contribute to optimism. Many of these people involved with making health care, disease prevention and control a positive undertaking arise every day planning to make life and living a little better for the less fortunate. Some have developed a "love affair" for their calling. This is cause for hope and optimism, even in a world of darkness – service to others is still deemed a priority by many dedicated to the advancement of

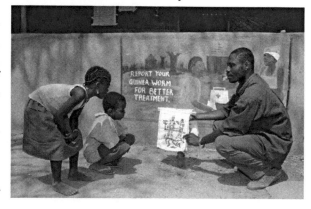

public health. Optimism can only be truly realized as an incontestable principle when no one in the world is denied medical care or treatment because he or she is too poor, regardless of the resource capability of the country. Is that a realistic expectation? That remains our collective challenge.

There is every reason to be optimistic, at least cautiously so, with the satisfying thought that the Bill and Melinda Gates Foundation will continue "being shrewd about doing good....and then daring the rest of us to follow." Their commitment to conquer the major diseases that devastate poor countries must be a source of comfort to every village, town, and country throughout the developing world. The focused agenda and professional commitment of the Carter Center in just about every facet of growth and development in the least developed countries, with emphasis on global health initiatives, provides cause for optimism. The dynamic humanitarianism of Doctors Without Borders, as interventionists, is reason for comfort. This organization has done so much excellent work that any attempt to describe or measure their accomplishments will not do justice to their unselfish outreach and success to make life more livable for the least fortunate and most in need among us.

The passion of former President William Jefferson Clinton and his active leadership of the Clinton Global Initiative to help people experience better tomorrows through outreach programs to establish a global community that will improve lives by alleviating poverty and introducing varied objectives for economic growth and development, including health promotion to influence change, is cause for optimism and hope. The William J. Clinton Foundation and the Clinton Global Initiative (CGI) will continue to be a part of global health policy in the future, and an agent for change to benefit mankind. The Earth Institute of Columbia University with Jeffrey Sachs and his colleagues, is an ideal example how the academic community could influence the collective effort to provide critical infrastructure to fight disease and help the poorest of the poor move to another tier towards a better life through economic growth and development, and that utopian dream – the end of poverty.

The developed countries have historically been able to provide essential public health services – the monitoring and surveillance of disease, the promotion of health, enforcement of public health laws and regulations, the administration of immunization programs, maintaining a public health infrastructure, and researching innovative solutions to health hazards of their populations. In contrast, the poor countries have been unable to develop and institute sustainable health services. It is more than the availability of clean water. It is about disease transmitting vectors like mosquitoes, uncollected garbage, sewage, no latrines, underemployment and limited to no jobs, environmental hazards, malnutrition and hunger, and an excessive prevalence of diseases of every category – infectious, chronic, and nutritional. It is about loss of hope, and no time to dream. It is about a paucity of money and inequality. It is also about the need for immediate action to correct the existing wrongs and deficits that would open windows of opportunity for living with dignity.

The health problems and challenges of the developing countries remain so overwhelming that ideas and ideals continue to be only vaguely apprehensible, frustrating optimism. Collective responses with technical and financial support will be needed to address and overcome the inequities for decades. The road ahead is long and arduous for the people themselves, the governments, foundations and organizations, demanding concerted efforts to achieve a semblance of hope or optimism. Poverty and social injustice will continue to be deterrents, even in developed countries. Despite the "darkness," developing countries cannot afford to indulge in the negatives and barriers they face. They still, as a unified group, have to make strategic prioritizations for the future to eradicate the burden of poverty, promote education and health, pursue sound environmental practices, and establish systems for social and economic development.

Social justice is an inherent part of the soul of every nation. It is a source of internal strength that is necessary to progress and succeed. It cannot be promoted or created for countries – it has to be integral to the thinking, policies and philosophy of individual governments. It heightens cooperation, collaboration, and accountability, and provides hope and optimism for fairness and equity. Thus, as we re-examine the original question, whether or not there is reason for optimism, the answer remains difficult. But, optimism and hope will prevail, with tremendous sacrifices and collectivity, if we are willing to help eliminate the blight of poverty, improve the standard of living and health care, and promote the dignity of humanity. It will not happen any time soon. We have to build a long-term vision for optimism and hope, with a lot of faith and charity, if we have any hope to succeed. Support of the Millennium Development Goals (MDGs), our current reason for optimism, is encouraged, whether or not some of the objectives will be realized or not. At least, it is another attempt to look forward and amplify optimism.

Since living mandates that we look beyond the dark clouds of negatives and seek hope and optimism for the future of the developing countries, we must not forget, nonetheless, that we live in a world where a billion people live on less than $1 a day, and ubiquitous poverty continues to be the most pressing public health challenge, in spite of the many traditional assistance programs which have failed. Global public health core mission must be to eliminate poverty, protect the environment, heighten sustainable food production, and promote social and economic development and health equity as objectives. We have absolutely no choice but to join hands under difficult circumstances and challenging conditions to assure a better life for the underprivileged and use optimism as a guiding light. In fact, optimism is not an option, it is an imperative.

"It is our responsibility as health workers to respect human rights and to regard a person's dignity as foremost in the practice of our profession in order to impact quality of life – from the miraculous dawn to its sunset."

Manuel Velasco Suarez, 1914-2001

Don A. Franco

"Health is a crossroads. It is where biological and social factors, the individual and the community, and social and economic policy all meet. In addition to having its own intrinsic value, health is a means toward personal and collective realization; it is therefore also an index of the success achieved by a society and its government institutions in the search for well-being, which after all, is the ultimate goal of development."

Julio Frenk, Dean, Harvard School of Public Health

Epilogue

Reflections of the past make it clear that we have to do better in the future by providing a more realistic vision and, hopefully, better rational objectives to guide a new path to the progress of global health, especially in the least developed countries of the planet. We are presently living in the throes of global health at the crossroads with a demanding imperative for a renewed sense of purpose to achieve needed changes that will make health care services and interventions more accessible to the poor of the world. The United States Declaration of Independence in 1776 addressed life, liberty, and the pursuit of happiness as thematic for the country's aspirations. The formatting of the Universal Declaration of Human Rights in 1948 recognized the dignity of the human family and the right to a standard of living that is adequate for the health and well-being of people, and the necessity for social protection, including the principles of common values to respect freedom.

In 1978 in Alma-Ata, Russia (now Kazakhstan), a global health coalition, organized and supported by the World Health Organization, enthusiastically affirmed that access to basic health services was a fundamental right and that "health for all" by the year 2000, using the principles of primary health care would improve ways to prevent diseases, contribute to a better standard of living, and enhance health objectives, especially among the vulnerable poor of the world. In spite of the idealism and rightness of the program, the concept, principles, and objectives were not accomplished within the projected timeframe, and, sadly, must be deemed a failure. In the establishment of the goals, limitations were overlooked, and hyper-inflation of what was projected to be possible to achieve exceeded reality, contributing to the lack of accomplishments and the obvious resulting disappointment. Basically, we had great dreams clashing with reality.

The lack of any measurable success of the "health for all 2000" program provided impetus for the global health leadership of the

United Nations, through its arm, the World Health Organization, to conduct an intensive self-examination of the whys of failure. This was a difficult process, but it took a form of immediacy when it was recognized that there was no way to salvage the program in the midst of severe criticism and ridicule from many different sectors who initially thought the objectives were unduly too ambitious. Not to be outdone in any future planning, the United Nations quickly sought a new initiative, with more comprehensive and defined intervention strategies. In September 2000, at its New York headquarters, the UN adopted another broad set of renewed goals defined as the Millennium Development Goals (MDGs) within a Millennium Declaration that prioritized social and economic improvements and national development, in general, in the less developed countries, with a timeframe to be achieved by the year 2015 (Refer to Chapter 3). Unfortunately, the interim assessments measuring the progress of the MDGs have been less than encouraging, especially in the poorest sectors of the world, indicating the likelihood of another disappointing WHO/UN declaration. Credit must be given to the successes of some of the goals, but considered as a unit, the MDGs fell short of expectations. The MDGs could be considered another example of hyper-inflationary objectives. The euphoria about doing good and contributing to the relief of poor masses throughout the world is exemplary, but must be done within the constraints of the possible.

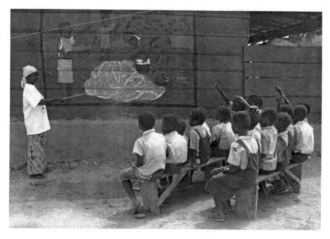

Water, sanitation, and hygiene (WASH) and the relevance to health are as old as civilization and will remain a collective and compelling challenge to global health for decades in all countries. Their deficits will become especially acute, and an ongoing affront to public health in resource challenged countries. The fact that 40 percent of people worldwide, exemplified by the poor countries, have no access to toilets and adequate sanitation and hygiene demonstrate the monstrous problem for public health. Infectious diseases, comparatively well-managed and prevented and controlled in industrialized countries, will continue to be an excessive burden for developing countries. Interestingly, and a challenge to all countries, is the emergence of new microbes, especially many of zoonotic pertinence. Additionally, antibiotic resistance would become a complicating factor for the prevention and control of infectious diseases for many decades, likely forever. Developing countries will have an additional burden to invest in capacity building if there is going to be any hope to respond effectively to the continuing onslaught of the excessive disease prevalence, both infectious and chronic, that exists in their regions of the world.

Chronic diseases have become the leading cause of mortality in the world, representing more than 60 percent of all deaths or about 35 million people annually. Heart disease, stroke, cancer, chronic respiratory diseases and diabetes are the major causes of the deaths. The fact that people are living longer in all spheres of the globe, with the exception of sub-Saharan Africa whose populations have been devastated by HIV/AIDS, affirms new dimensions and challenges for chronic diseases. Research in the past three decades that has demonstrated microbial agents as a complex and link to chronic diseases amplifies the burden and the necessity to look at new options to address the epidemiology and control/prevention of chronic diseases.

Hunger and malnutrition continue to be at the epicenter of the public health debate, and begs the logical question, what policies are necessary to contribute to needed reforms that will positively impact the developing countries, especially those that are least developed and most at risk? Poverty is the principle cause of hunger and malnutrition and there is no hope that there could be any progress or improvements without the alleviation/elimination of it, as a social injustice. This will be dependent on a change in the socio-economic status of resource-burdened countries and the populations that inhabit them. The thought, however, that one sixth of the world's population live on $1 or less a day provides little solace or hope for change. Whether or not the concept of sustainable food production could be incorporated into national development programs of resource-poor countries is now a part of the debating options. Can this initiative ever be viewed and pursued as a public health imperative to help alleviate hunger and malnutrition and other aspects of poverty? That will have to be determined by the political leadership, and the collective will of the people. It is worthy, however, of serious consideration, because the potential long term benefits, if properly and successfully implemented, are enormous to societies in poor countries.

The challenges for public health in developing countries could be rationally combined with some of the considerations whether or not there is any cause for optimism. Acceptance that 60 to 75 percent of people in the developing countries still lack access to basic primary health care is reason for serious concern. A nation's well-being and health is dependent on nutritional programs, a good public health infrastructure, promotion and support of basic healthcare programs, education as a political priority, and proper maintenance of a healthy environment.

Optimism must be linked to realism, and as we examine the burdensome challenges that global health strategists face, we can also study the happenings of the present to determine whether or not there is really a cause for hope. Using Haiti as reality and a comparative base, we can obtain a sense of the problems of poverty, hunger, disease and health from the broadest perspective and analyze whether or not we have met the basic responsibilities, indeed, accountabilities of a successful response to their plight as a people. After all, whether or not we want to accept it, the globe is made up of many countries that simulate Haiti, and it is not unreasonable to make the tragedies that the country experienced a model for analysis and evaluation of outcomes. And, that is the reason for going beyond what an epilogue is normally meant to accomplish. I seek understanding for my liberties in doing so. An epilogue is meant to be a final note or summary, and not a discourse for extensive discussion. Nonetheless, I wanted to make Haiti metaphorically applicable to other less developed countries and see whether or not we can follow a path of lessons learned to evaluate the successes or failures of outcomes, considerate of a global health context. Hopefully, Haiti can become a memory for other interventions. If we do not remember the past, we may be condemned to repeat it. The failures in Haiti were symptomatic of mass confusion, no governance, official dysfunction, and institutional failures.

Haiti's earthquake occurred on January 12, 2010, causing major and catastrophic damage in the capital of Port-au-Prince and contiguous regions of the country. Three million people were affected by the earthquake, out of a population of 9.7 million, of which more than 1,000,000 million are still homeless today, and an estimated 230,000 dead. Just about every continent and country reached out to Haiti. The humanitarian response was cause for gratitude. People, in times of calamity show their best. The United States, ever prepared to assist those in need was, as expected and customary, a first responder. The country also mobilized former President Bill Clinton as a special United Nations envoy to coordinate and assist the compelling relief efforts. His mere presence and outreach was a source of inspiration in an atmosphere of chaotic hopelessness and total turmoil. As of this writing (November 27, 2010), about 80% of the rubble from the quake has not been cleared, because of the lack of infrastructure and governance, caused by the indignity of poverty. The temporary "camps" used for housing the displaced had no water or sewage disposal, no electricity. Disorganized chaos, discontent, the void of leadership prevailed and there was a total lack of any form of protection of the people from the post-ravages of the disaster. Poor government = poor to no resources = inability to respond = widespread confusion = fear = no civic order = the will and commitment of the heroic few could not be sustained = breakdown in law and order = no one knowing anything about anything! The poorest of the poor in the poorest country of the Western hemisphere trying to merely survive in a maze of uncertainty, heightened by the continuing fear of more uncertainty!

There was heightened concern and fear that the deplorable living conditions following the earthquake would result in disease outbreaks. All the cumulative threatening hazards to health pointed to the likelihood that an infectious disease like cholera was only a matter of time. The trepidation became a reality when people started displaying signs of diarrhea and other symptoms simulating cholera in early October. This was later positively confirmed by a definitive diagnosis of cholera on October 21, 2010. It is of interest to note that Haiti, in spite of its widespread poverty, has not had a diagnosed case of cholera for decades. The acuteness of the disease challenge and the fear of global health experts was that in the capital city of Port-au-Prince, a population of about 3 million people, about half were already living in temporary encampments. Rapid spread of the cholera with high mortality linked to the consequences and circumstances of the earthquake, the displaced people, and the close to total collapse of the country's health care system was reason for serious concern. The overcrowding, lack of organization and coordination of services, shortage of professional staff and supplies, contributed to widespread discontent and alarm with many patients having to be treated in the streets, among the rising death toll,

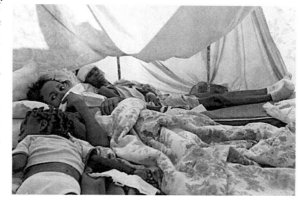

approximating over 1600 (November 28, 2010). No one seemed fully in charge or in control because of the paucity of governance and the utter impossibility of it all since the earthquake. Protests and a complete breakdown of law and order followed. The fear of death became a constant. People lacked faith that anything good can happen. Many wondered why a poor country like Haiti had to be subjected to so many calamitous events – one after another. Anger became a response mechanism, and young men started to throw rocks and threaten United Nations personnel. There was increased anger and more fear. Sadness and a sense of hopelessness were evident, but many Haitians were still able to maintain a resiliency that defies explanation, in spite of being helpless. Children smiled and played in the rubble with hope, many not understanding the immensity of the disaster. Bureaucratic blunders and indifference did not help. This forced Doctors Without Borders, a well-known international health organization to express frustration, unusual for this body, by issuing a public statement saying that in spite of the presence of an overabundance of international organizations, the responses came nowhere close to meeting the needs of the people.

While there are no guarantees that using the calamitous happenings in Haiti as any form of indicator or guideline for helping or predicting in the future, there are distinct lessons that international organizations like the United Nations can learn from and hopefully apply to other relief efforts including global health initiatives. Global health policies aspire to lofty goals and principles, but our implementation methods are somewhat imperfect and definitely suspect as we examine the historical record. The Universal Declaration of Human Rights, "Health for All by the year 2000," the Millennium Development Goals, Alleviation of Hunger, Malnutrition and Poverty, Disease Control and Prevention – are all most worthy aspirations. Yet, we continue to stumble over the hurdles, and approach forks in the road and not recognize the warnings!

There is, nonetheless, still every reason for hope and optimism despite the depressing problems that the resource poor countries face daily. When one witnesses the unselfish reaching out of individuals, small groups, the religious working in missions and hospitals, the efforts of so many in national governments and world bodies, and the active involvement of foundations and organizations dedicated to helping people live better and healthier....there is every reason to be hopeful and optimistic. That is not a choice. It is what we must do for the art of betterment and the uplifting of humanity's less fortunate.

Global inequalities will likely continue for many years and the problems will remain tenuous, demanding, and fraught with obstacles, necessitating a collective will of global brotherhood and humanitarianism if we have any hope to alleviate and eliminate one day the throes of poverty and the concomitant affront to global public health which approximates a crisis today. The only thing that we have left is optimism. We are bound by decency and our obligations to the world's needy to be participants and advocates for change. That is part of a civilized global society and life in a contracted world where we are so dependent on each other in our quest of improving the lot of humanity.

"The challenges ahead are great, but the world has never been in a better position to drastically improve global health. We have the tools to prevent many of the worst diseases; we have the scientific knowledge to develop new solutions; and we have growing political commitment and resources.

"Working together, we can save millions of lives, and change the world's view of what's possible."
www.changingthepresent.org/global_health

"You cannot tackle hunger, disease, and poverty unless you can also provide people with a healthy ecosystem in which their economies can grow."

Dr. Gro Harlem Brundtland, Former Director-General, WHO

"We started our foundation because we believe we have a real opportunity to help advance equity around the world....to help make sure that, no matter where a person is born, he or she has the chance to live a healthy, productive life."
Melinda Gates, Bill and Melinda Gates Foundation

References and Notes

Introduction

• Facts on World Hunger and Poverty. Publication of statistics citing major international organizations like UNICEF, WHO, the World Bank, World Food Program, and FAO Hunger Report. www.heartandminds.org/poverty/hungerfactes.htm.

• United Methodist Committee on Relief (UMCOR) – Facts About World Hunger/Poverty. New York, N.Y. 10115.

• Moyo, D. 2009. Dead Aid: Why Aid Is Not Working And How There Is A Better Way For Africa. Farrar, Straus, and Giroux. New York.

• Easterly, W. 2007. The White Man's Burden. Penguin Books, London.

• Yunus, M. 2003. Banker to the Poor. Public Affairs, N.Y.

• Franco, D. 2009. Poverty and the Continuing Global Health Crisis. Tate Publishing & Enterprises. Mustang, OK.

• The National Academic Press. 1997. America's Vital Interest in Global Health: Protecting Our People, Financing Our Economy, and Advancing Our International Interests.

Chapter 1

• Universal Declaration of Human Rights. A United Nations Priority. http://un.org/rights/HRToday/declar.htm

• The History of the Bill of Rights. Human Rights. The pursuit of an ideal. http://thinkquest.org/C0126065/billhistory.html

• The Universal Declaration of Human Rights. http://un.org.en/documents/udhr

• The United States Declaration of Independence. http://wikipedia.org/wiki/United_States_Declaration

• Declaration of the Rights of Man and of the Citizen. http://en.wikipedia.org

• World Health Organization. Progress report by the Lancet of remarks by Dr. Margaret Chan, Director-General of the World Health Organization on Return to Alma-Ata outlining the guiding principles of primary health care articulated in 1978 during that initial declaration to organize the full range of health options. www.who.int/dg/20080915/en/index.html

• Franco, D.A.: 2007. Poverty ~ Malnutrition ~ Disease ~ Hopelessness: A Cry for Social Justice. Sierra Publishing, Camino, California.
• The National Academies Press. 1997. America's Vital Interest in Global Health: Protecting Our People, Financing Our Economy, and Advancing Our International Interests.
• Reid, T. R.: 2009. The Healing of America – A Global Quest For better, Cheaper, And Fairer Health Care. The Penguin Press. New York.
• World Health Organization. The World Health Report 2008. Primary Health Care – Now More Than Ever. ISBN 978 92 4 156373 4.
• Michael Tomasky: Healthcare vote: Barack Obama passes US health reform by narrow margin – guardian.co.uk. March 22, 2010. (This article by Tomasky was referenced to get a sense of the reaction from the United Kingdom that has a universal health coverage system that has been highlighted in discussions during the Congressional debate).
• Farmer, P.: 2005. Pathologies of Power. Health, Human Rights, and the New War on the Poor. University of California Press, Berkeley.
• Neill, K. G.: 2000. Dancing with the Devil: Health, Human Rights, and the Export of U.S. Models of Managed Care to Developing Countries. www.culturalsurvival.org/ourpublication/csp/article/dancing-with-devil-health-hum...
• Rosenberg, M.L., E.S. Hayes, M.H. McIntyre, and N. Neill: 2010. Real Collaboration – What It Takes for Global Health to Succeed. University of California Press, Berkeley.

Chapter 2

• Valentine, V.: 2005. Health for the Masses: China's "Barefoot Doctors" – www.npr.org/templates/story/story.php/storyId-4990242

• Zhang, D. and P.U. Unschuld: 2008. China's barefoot doctor: past, present, and future: The Lancet, Volume 372, Issue 9653, pgs. 1865-1867. http:www.lancet.com/journals/lancet/article/PHS0140-6736(08)61355-0/fulltext?_eventld..

• Franco, D.A.: 2009. Poverty and the Continuing Global Health Crisis. Tate Publishing & Enterprises. Mustang, Oklahoma.

• Habicht, J.P.: 1981. Health for All by the Year 2000. Amer. Jour. Pub. Hlth. Vol. 71, No. 5. Pgs. 459-461.

• Hall, J.J. and R. Taylor.: 2003. Health for all beyond 2000: the demise of the Alma-Ata Declaration and primary health care in developing countries. MJA, Vol. 178. Pgs. 17-20.

• International Policy Network. Diseases of Poverty and the 10/90 gap. In an article written by Philip Stevens, Director of Health Projects (2004) of the Policy Network, the author described the neglected diseases and the association to poverty in lower income countries. (International Policy Network, Third Floor, Bedford Chambers, The Piazza, London WC2E 8HA UK). www.fightingdiseases.org/pdf/Diseases

• Institute of Medicine. The Infectious Etiology of Chronic Diseases – Defining the Relationship, Enhancing the research, and Mitigating the Effects. Workshop Summary. The National Academies Press, Washington, D.C. 2004.

• Health for All by the Year 2000 – its Foundation and Future. www.portfolio.mvm.ed.ac.uk/studentswebs/sessionl/group76/jane page.htm

• Morley, D., J. Rohde, and G. Williams.: 1983. Practicing Health for All. Oxford. Oxford Medical Publications.

Chapter 3

• http://en.wikipedia.org/wiki/Millennium_Development_G oals

• www.un.org/millenniumgoals/bkgd.shtml

• Sen, A.: 1999. Development as Freedom. Random House, Inc., New York.

- Garrett, L.: 2000. Betrayal of Trust: The Collapse of Global Public Health. Hyperion, New York.
- Franco, D.A.: 2009. Poverty and the Continuing Global Health Crisis. Tate Publishing and Enterprises, Mustang, Oklahoma.
- "After 2015: Rethinking Pro-Poor Policy" (www.ids.ac.uk/download.cfm/file=IF9.1.pdf) Institute of Development Studies (IDS) In Focus Policy Brief 9.1. June 2009.
- Perkins, A.: 2008. Time to review the development goals, guardian.co.uk. (In a provocative article in the Guardian (U.K.) when government leaders from throughout the world were meeting in New York to discuss the progress of the Millennium Development Goals (MDGs), Ms Perkins presented the widespread problems and challenges faced by many countries that appear unable to achieve the goals).
- Shah, A.: Causes of Poverty. http://globalissues.org/TradeRelated/Poverty.asp.
- The World Bank Group. Millennium Development Goals. http://ddp-ext.worldbank.org/ext/GMS/gms.do/silted
- Seager, A.: 2010. Recession is crippling hope for universal primary education UN warns. www.guardian.co.uk/education/2010/jan/20/education-for-allo-unesco-wanring
- Study says universal education is attainable and affordable. www.voanews.com/english/archive/2007-01/2007-01-17-voa83.
- Stiglitz, J.E.: 2007. Making Globalization Work. W. W. Norton & Company, N.Y., New York.
- United Nations. End Poverty 2015 – Fact Sheet. Department of Public Information – DPI/25171 – September 2008.
- http://en.wikipedia.org/wiki/Gender_equality
- UNICEF: Millennium Development Goals: 3. Promote gender equality and empower women. http://unicef.org/gener/index_25492.html.
- www.medterms.com/script/main/art.asp
- UNICEF Data Shows Global Child Deaths Now Below 9 M Annually, Progress Not Enough To Achieve MDG In Most Regions. http://medicalnewstoday.com/articles/163680.php

- National Center for Policy Analysis. Health Issues. Study Finds Big Decrease in Global Child Mortality. www.ncpa.org/sub/dpd/index.php
- WHO. Maternal mortality falling too slowly to meet goal. http://who.int/mediacentre/new/releases/2007/pr56/en/index.html
- Medical News Today. Study Shows Progress On Global Maternal Mortality. www.medicalnewstoday.com/articles/185500.php
- The White Ribbon Alliance for Safe Motherhood. Global Maternal Fact Sheet. www.MotherDayEveryDay.org
- The Global Fund to Fight AIDS, Tuberculosis, and Malaria. www.avert.org/global-fund.htm
- U.S. Global Health Policy. www.globalhealthfacts.org
- ww.one.org/aids_poverty
- A History of Tuberculosis. http://state.nj.us/health/cd/tbhistry.htm
- History of Malaria: Scientific Discoveries. http://malariasite.com/malaria/history_science.htm
- Department of Economic and Social Affairs. Statistics Division. Progress towards the Millennium Development Goals, 1990-2005. http://unstats.un.org/unsd/mi/goals_2005/goal_...
- World Health Organization. 1996. The State of World Health. In the World Health Report 1996 – Fighting disease, fostering development. 1-62. Geneva.
- Environment and human well-being: a practical strategy. UN Task Force on Environmental Sustainability. http://unmillenniumproject.org/document..
- UNDP. Millennium Development Goals. www.undp.org/mdg/progress.shtml
- Millennium Development Goals. Goal 8. Develop a Global Partnership for Development. www.undg.org/archive_docs/4532-Netherlands_MDG8
- Africa and the Millennium Development Goals. 2007. Update. www.un.org
- World Health Organization. 2007. Fact Sheet. No. 104.

Chapter 4

- Water and human health. Water as a global resource. http://openlearn.open.ac.uk/mod/resource/view.php/id=293806
- The World's Water. www.worldwater.org/data.20082009
- Global Policy Forum. http://globalpolicy.org/images/pdfs/troubled_water-complete.pdf
- http://waterfootprint.org/pagefiles/WaterFootprintsNations
- Centers for Disease Control and Prevention/Global Water, Sanitation & Hygiene (WASH) www.cdc.gov/healthywater/global
- Jesperson, K.: Search for Clean Water Continues. www.nesc.wvu.edu/old_website/ndwc_DWH_1.html
- Hu, H. and N.H. Kim. 1003. Drinking Water Pollution and Human Health. In Critical Condition: Human Health and the Environment, eds. E. Chivian, E. Haines, H. Hu, and M. McCally, 31-48, Cambridge; Massachusetts Institute of Technology Press.
- Public Health at a Glance, Water, Sanitation & Hygiene. http://web.worldbank.org/WBSITE/EXTERNAL/TOPICS/EXTHALT...
- United Nations University, Institute for Water, Environment and Health. 2010. Sanitation as a Key to Global Health: Voices from the Field. ISBN: 92-808-6012-7
- World Health Organization. 1996. The World Health Report 1996. Fighting disease, fostering development,27-39. Geneva. WHO
- Okun, D.A. 1992. Water Quality Management. In Maxcy-Rosenau-Last Public Health and Preventive Medicine, 13th Edition, eds. J.M. Last and R.B. Williams, 619-648. Norwalk, CT: Appleton and Lange.
- de Silva, N.R., S. Brooker, P.J. Hotez, A. Montresor, D. Engles, and L. Savioli. 2003. "Soil-Transmitted Helminth Infections: Updating the Global Picture." Trends in Parasitology 19: 547-551.
- WHO. Water, sanitation and hygiene links to health. www.who.int/water_sanitation_health/publications/facts2004/en/
- WHO. What is guinea worm? www.who.int/features/ga/14/en/index/html

Don A. Franco

• Spencer, H.C.: 1991. Dracunculiasis. In Hunter's Tropical Medicine, ed. G.T. Strickland, 750-756. Philadelphia. W.B. Saunders Co.

• Centers for Disease Control and Prevention. Division of Parasitic Diseases. Fact Sheet. Dracunculiasis. www.cdc.gov/NCIDOD/DPD/parasites/dracunculiasis/factsht_dra cunculiasis.htm

• Eddleston, M., R. Davidson, R. Wilkinson and S. Pierini (eds.) 2005. Trachoma. Oxford Handbook of Tropical Medicine, 2nd ed. Oxford University Press, N.Y. 482-483.

• WHO. Malaria. www.who.int/mediacentre/factsheets/fs094/en/

• Hadler, S.C.: 1991. Global impact of hepatitis A virus infection changing patterns. In Viral Hepatitis and Liver Diseases, eds. F.B. Hollinger, S.M. Lemon, and H.S. Morgalis, 214. Baltimore, Williams and Wilkins.

• Lemon, S.M. and S.P. Day. 1991. Type A Viral Hepatitis. In Infectious Diseases, eds. S.L. Gorbach, J.G. Bartlett, and N.R. Blacklow. 705-709. Philadelphia, W.B. Saunders Co.

• WHO. Aresnic, drinking-water and health risk substitution in arsenic mitigation. www.who.int/water_sanitation_health/dwq/wsh0306/en/index.htm l

• NRDC: Arsenic in Drinking Water. www.nrdc.org/water/drinking/qarsenic.asp

• T. Kjellstrom et al. Air and Water pollution: Burden and Strategies for Control. In Disease Control Priorities in Developing Countries. 2nd Edition. D.T. Jamison, J.G. Breman, A.R. Mearsham, G. Alleyne, M. Claeson, D.B. Evans, P. Jha, A. Miller, and P. Musgrave. Eds. 817-832. The International Bank for Reconstruction and Development/The World Bank, Washington, D.C.

• http://medical-dictionary.thefreedictionary.com/fluorosis

• WHO. Water-related diseases. www.who.int/water_sanitation_health/diseases/fluorosis/en/

• WHO. Poor sanitation threatens public health. www.who.int/mediacentre/news/releases/2008/pr08/en/index.html

• Disease and sanitation. http://tilz.tearfund.org/Publications/Footsteps+1=10Footsteps+9Disease..

• Rosenberg, C.E. 1992. Explaining Epidemics and Other Studies in the History of Medicine. 109-121. Cambridge University Press.

Chapter 5

• Monto, A.S., and C.F. Marrs. 1997. Infectious Agents. In Oxford Textbook of Public Health, 3rd ed. Vol. 1., eds. R. Detels, W.W. Holland, J. McEwen, and G.S. Omenn. 175-198. New York: Oxfor University Press.

• Kaas, A.M. and E.H. Kass. 1992. A Perspective on the History of Infectious Diseases, eds. S.L. Gorbach, J.G. Bartlett, and N.R. Blacklow, 1-6. Philadelphia: W.B. Saunders Co.

• The Enlightenment and its impact on medicine. www.rcseng.ac.uk/museums/exhibiting_difference/learning/resource_pack/The Enlightenment and medicine.pdf

• The Enlightenment. http://facuty.ucc.edu/egh-damerow/the_enlightenment.htm

• Biography of Antony van Leeuwenhoek. http://www.essortment.com/all/biographyantony_rcoc.htm

• Anthony van Leeuwenhoek (1632-1723) www.ucmp.berkeley.edu/history/leeuwenhoek.html

• Edward Jenner (1749-1823) www.zephyrus.co.uk/edwardjenner.html

• History of Antiseptics – Ignaz Semmelweis http://inventors.com/library/inventors/blantiseptics,htm

• Ignaz Philipp Semmelweis (1818-1865) http://cdc.gov/ncidod/eid/vol/no2cover.htm

• Louis Pasteur – Wikipedia, the free encyclopedia. http://en.wikipedia.org/wiki/Louis_Pasteur

• Louis Pasteur (1822-1895) www.accessexcellence.org/RC/AB/BC/Louis_Pasteur.php

• Lamont, A.: 1992. Joseph Lister: father of modern surgery. Creation 14 (2): 48-51. www.answersingenesis.org/creation/v14/12/scientists,asp

- www.referencecenter.com/ref/reference/Koch_Rob/Rober t_Koch/invocationType+ar1clk&tflv=1
- www.nndb.com/people/618/000091345/
- http://myhero.com/go/print/asp/hero=robert_koch
- www.faqs.org/health/bios/13Robert-Koch.html
- http://en.wikipedia.org/wiki/Pual_Ehrlich
- http://nobelprize.org/nobel_prizes/medicine/laureates/1908/ehrlich-bio.html
- www.whonamedit.com/doctor.cfm/696.html
- http://answers.com/topic/hans-christian-gram
- www.rsc.org/chemistryworld/Issues/2010/February/Petri
- www.hoslink.com/history2.htm#petrie
- www.epidemic.org/theFacts/viruses/theOriginsOfViruses.php
- www.bookrags.com/biography/dmitri-iosifovich-ivanovsky-wmi
- http://en.academic.ru/dic.nsf/enwiki/114332
- www.apsnet.org/education/feature/tmv/intro.html
- http://en.wikipedia.org/wiki/Martinus_Beijernick
- http://yellowfever.lib.virginia.edu/reed/reed.html
- www.brittanica.com/EBchecked/topic/494983/Walter_Reed
- http://en.wikipedia.org/wiki/Yellow_fever
- http://nobelprize.org/nobel_prizes/medicine/laureates/1945/fleming-bio.html
- www.sjsu.edu/depts/Museum/flemin.html
- www.referencecenter.com/ref/reference/FlemingA/Sir_Alexander_
- www.en.wikipedia.org/wiki/DNA_sequencing
- www.genomenewsnetwork.org/resources/timeline/1977_Gilbert.php
- www.medterms.com/script/main/art.asp/articlekey=4807
- http://science.howstuffworks.com/dictionary/famous-science/biologists
- www.karymullis.com/biography.shtml
- www.accessexcellence.org/WN/SUA06/hflu.php
- http://archievesciencewatch.com/jan-feb2002_page3.htm

• Thro, E.: 1993. Genetic Engineering – Shaping the Material of Life. Facts on File, Inc. New York, N.Y.
• http://sandwalk.blogspot.com/2008/10/nobel-laureate-stanley-prusiner.html
• www.brittanica.com/EBchecked/topic/480887/Stanley-B-Prusiner
• Franco, D.A., 2005. An Introduction to the Prion Diseases of Animals: Assessing the History, Risk Inferences, and Public Health Implications in the United States. The National Renderers Association. ISBN 0-9654660-2-7
• www.jewishvirtuallibrary.org/source/biography/prusiner.html
• Franco, D.A.: 2007. Poverty ~ Malnutrition ~ Disease ~ Hopelessness: A Cry for Social Justice. Sierra Publishing, Camino, California.
• Institute of Medicine. 2003. Microbial Threats to Health. The National Academies Press, Washington, D.C.
• Morse, S.S.: 1995. Factors in the Emergence of Infectious Diseases. Emerging Infectious Diseases. Vol. 1, Number 1, January-March, 1995. www.cdc.gov/ncidod/eid/vol1no1/morse.htm
• Fauci, A.S. 2006. 2005 Robert H. Ebert Memorial Lecture – Emerging and Re-emerging Infectious Diseases: The Perpetual Challenge. www.milbank.org/reports/0601farci.html
• Taylor, L.H., S.M. Latham, and M.E. Woodhouse. 2001. Risk Factors for Human Disease Emergence. Philosophical Transactions of the Royal Society B: Biological Sciences 356: 983-89.
• Weiss, R.A. and A.J. McMichael: 2004. Social and environmental risk factors in the emergence of infectious diseases. Nature Medicine 10, 870-876. www.nature.com/nm/journal/v10/nl2s/full/nml150.hml
• Cutler, S.J, A.R. Fooks, and W.H.M. van der Poel: 2010. Public Health Threat of New, Reemerging, and Neglected Zoonoses in the Industrialized World. Emerging Infectious Diseases. Vol. 6. No 1. 1-7. www.cdc.gov/eid. Vol. 16. No 1, January 2010.

Don A. Franco

Chapter 6

- WHO. Preventing Chronic Diseases A Vital Investment. www.who.int/chp/chronic_disease_report/contents/partl.pdf
- Finch, C.E. and E.L. Schneider. 1996. Biology of Aging. In Cecil Textbook of Medicine. 2oth ed., eds. J.C. Bennett and F. Plum, 12-15. Philadelphia: W.B. Saunders Co.
- Luepker, R.V. 2002. Cardiovascular Diseases. In Oxford Textbook of Public Health, 4th ed., eds. R. Detels, J. McEwen, R. Beaglehole, and H. Tanaka, 1127-1154. New York: Oxford University Press.
- Institute of Medicine. 2004. The Infectious Etiology of Chronic Diseases. Washington, D.C.: The National Academies Press.
- Berkow, R., ed. 2005. Neoplasms. In the Merck Veterinary Manual, 9th ed. 2248-2255.
- www.gsksource.com/gskprm/en/US/adirect/gskprm/cmd= Product
- http://en.wikipedia.org/wiki/HPV_vaccine
- Franco, E.L.: 2004. The Role of Viruses in Oncogenesis: Human Papillomaviruses and cervical Cancer as a Paradigm. In the Infectious Etiology of Chronic Diseaes. Eds. S. Knobler, S. O'Connor, S.M. Lemon, and M. Najafi. 17-28. Washington, D.C.: National Academies Press.
- Malawista, S.E.: 1996. Lyme Disease. In Cecil Textbook of Medicine, 20th ed., eds. J.C. Bennett and F. Plum. 1715-1720. Philadelphia: W.B. Saunders Co.
- Mason, W.: 2004. Chronic Hepatitis B Virus Infections. In the Infectious Etiology of Chronic Diseases, eds. S. Knobler, S. O'Connor, S.M. Lemon, and M. Najafi, 28-35. Washington, D.C. National Academies Press.
- Krieger, N.: 1994. Epidemiology and the web of causation. Has anyone seen the spider? Social Science and Medicine. 39: 887.
- Centers for Disease Control and Prevention. Chronic Disease Prevention. www.cdc.gov/nccdphp

- Beaglehole, R. and D. Yach. 2003. Globalization and the prevention and control of non-communicable disease: the neglected chronic diseases of adults. The Lancet 362: 903-908.
- Ferlay, J., F. Bray, P. Pisani, and D.M. Parkin. 2001. Globocan 2000: cancer incidence, mortality and prevalence worldwide. IARC Cancer Base No 5, Lyon, France: International Agency for Research on Cancer.
- Boffetta, P., P. Brennan, and R. Saracci. 2002. Neoplasms. In Oxford Textbook of Public Health, 4th ed., eds. R. Detels, J. McEwen, R. Beaglehole, and H. Tanaka. 1155-1192. New York: Oxford University Press.
- Yach, D. 2006. Chronic Diseases. In Social Injustice and Public Health, eds. B.S. Levy and V.W. Sidel, 253-276. New York: Oxford University Press.
- World Health Organization. 1996. The World Health Report 1996 – Fighting disease/Fostering development. The state of world health. Geneva: World Health Organization.
- Lam, T.H., and A. J. Hedley. 2002. Respiratory disease. In Oxford Textbook of Public Health. 4th ed., eds. R. Detels, J. McEwen, R. Beaglehole, and H. Tanaka. 1227-1254. New York: Oxford University Press.
- King, H., R.E. Aubert, and W.H. Herman. 1998. Global burden of diabetes, 1995-2025: prevalence, numerical estimates, and projections. Diabetes Care 21: 1414-1431.
- Wild, S., G. Roglic, A. Green et al. 2004. Global prevalence of diabetes: estimates for 2000 and projections for 3030. Diabetes Care 27: 1047-1053.
- Sherwin, R.S.: 1996. Diabetes Mellitus. In Cecil Textbook of Medicine, 20th ed., eds. J. C. Bennett and F. Plum, 1258-1277. Philadelphia: W.B. Saunders Co.
- Centers for Disease Control and Prevention. Global Health Activities. www2a.cdc.gov/od/gharview
- Centers for Disease Control and Prevention. www.cdc.gov/nccdphp/programs/globalhealth.htm
- McKeown, T.: 1991. The Origins of Human Disease. Oxford: Basil Blackwell Ltd.
- Sachs, J.D.: 2005. The End of Poverty: Economic Possibilities for Our Time. New York: The Penguin Press.

• Sartre, J.P.: 1971. Sketch for a Theory of the Emotions. London: Methuen.

Chapter 7

• Global Issues: World Hunger and Poverty Facts and Statistics 2010 www.worldhunger.org/articles/Learn/world hunger facts 2002.htm
• http://en.wikipedia.org/wiki?malnutrition
• Dreze, J. and A. Sen: 2002. Hunger and Public Action. Oxford University Press, Inc. New York.
• Shills, M.E. and V.R. Young, eds. 1988. Modern Nutrition in Health and Disease, 7th ed. Philadelphia: Lea and Febiger.
• Passmore, R. and M.A. Eastwood. 1986. Davidson and Passmore Human Nutrition and Dietetics ,, 8th ed. Edinburgh: Churchill-Livingstone.
• Nestle, K. 1992. Nutrition in Public Health and Preventive Medicine. In Marcy-Rosenau-Last Public Health and Preventive Medicine, eds. J.M. Last and R.B. Wallace, 995-1003. Norwalk, CT: Appleton and Lange.
• Shetty, P.S. and W.P.T. James. 1997. Nutrition. In Oxford Textbook of Public Health, 3rd. ed. Vol. 1 – The Scope of Public Health, eds. R. Detels, W.W. Holland, J. McEwen, and G.S. Omenn, 157-174. New York: Oxford University Press.
• www.unsystem.org/SCN/archives/nppl7/ch04.htm. Address by Hilde Frafjord Johnson, Minister of International Development and Human Rights (Norway) in Oslo, Norway, on the elimination of hunger and malnutrition.
• Scrimshaw, N.S. 1986. Nutrition and Preventive Medicine. In Maxcy-Rosenau Public Health and Preventive Medicine. 12th ed., ed. J.M. Last, 1515-1542. Norwalk, CT: Appleton-Century-Crofts.
• eMedicine. Marasmus. www.emedicine.com/ped/topic164.htm
• www.nlm.gov/medlineplus/ency/article/001604
• http://en.wikipedia.org.wiki/Kwashiorkor
• http://emedicine.medscape.com/article/126004-overview

• Berkow, R., M. H. Beers, and A.J. Fletcher, eds. 1997. Vitamins and Minerals. The Merck Manual of Medical Information. New York: Pocket Books
• www.anyvitamins.com/vitamin-b2-riboflavin-info.htm
• Roe, D.A. 1991. Pellagra – Nutritional Problems and Deficiency Diseases. In Hunter's Tropical Medicine, ed. G.T. Strickland, 932-934. Philadelphia: W.B. Saunders Co.
• www.cdc.gov/nutrition/everyone/basics/vitamins/iron.ht ml
• Khan, S.G. 1991. Iron Deficiency. Nutritional Problems and Deficiency Diseases. In Hunter's Tropical Medicine, ed. G. T. Strickland, 938-942. Philadelphia: W. B. Saunders Co.
• www.thyroid.org/patients/patient_brochures/iodine_defici ency.html
• Trowbridge, F.L. and J.B. Stanbury. 1991. Goiter and the Iodine Deficiency Disorders. In Hunter's Tropical Medicine, ed. G.T. Strickland, 942-945. Philadelphia: W.B. Saunders Co.
• World Hunger Education Service Associates. Hunger Notes – World Hunger Facts 2006. www.worldhunger.org/articles/Learn/world%20hunger%20facts% 202002.htm
• Brown, J.L. 2006. Nutrition. In Social Injustice and Public Health, eds. B.S. Levy and V.W. Sidel, 238-252. New York: Oxford University Press
• United Nations. 2006. Goal 1. Eradicate extreme poverty and hunger. The Millennium Development Goals Report 2006, p. 5.
• www.littlemag.com/hunger/swami.html

Chapter 8

• Food and Agriculture Organization of the United Nations. World agriculture 2030: Global food production will exceed population growth. www.fao.org/english/newsroom/news/2002/7828-en.html
• www.huffingtonpost.com/jose-w-fernandez/addressing-global-food

Don A. Franco

- Lianfu, L.: 1999. Development of sustainable food production and outlook. Agro-chemicals News in Brief. Special Issue, November 1999, 15-20.
- Anderson, P.P.: 2002. Towards a Sustainable Global Food System. What Will It Take? John Pesck Colloquium, Iowa State University, March 26-27, 2002. www.ifpri.org/pubs/articles/2002/pinstrup.
- Global Policy Forum. Hunger and the Globalized System of Trade and Food Production. www.globalpolicy.org/socecom/hunger/economy/index.htm
- Delgado, C.M., M. Rosegrant, H. Steinfeld, S. Ehui, and C. Courbois. 1999. Livestock to 2020. The Next Food Revolution. Report of a study coordinated by the International Food Policy Research Institute. Washington, D.C., Food and Agriculture Organization of the United Nations, Rome, and the International Livestock Research Institute, Nairobi, Kenya.
- World Health Organization. 1997. A New Perspective on Health. In health and Environment in Sustainable Development. Geneva. 1-17.
- Nestle, M.: 1992. Nutrition in Public Health and Preventive Medicine. In: Public Health and Preventive Medicine, eds. M.J. Last and R.B. Wallace. Appleton and Lange, Norwalk, CT. 995-1003.
- Austin, J.E.: 1981. Nutrition Programs in the Third World. Cases and Readings. Cambridge, MA.: Oelgeschlagen, Gunn, and Hain.
- Grant, J.P.: 1989. The State of the World's Children. New York. Oxford University Press (UNICEF).
- American Heritage Definition of Aquaculture.
- http://en.wikipedia.org/wiki/Aquaculture.
- Data extracted from the FAO Fisheries Global Aquaculture Database for freshwater crustaceans. 2005. The most recent data sets are for 2003 and reflect estimates.
- The Food and Agriculture Organization. Increasing food and agricultural production. www.nationencyclopedia.com?United-Nations-Related-Agencies

Chapter 9

- MacFarlane, S., M. Racelis, F. Muli-Muslime. 2000. The Lancet. Public health in developing countries. Volume 356. Issue 9232. 841-846.
- http://twas.ictp.it/news-in-home-page/news/health-in-transition
- Jamison, D.T., W. H. Mosley. 1991. American Journal of Public Health. Disease Control Priorities in Developing Countries: Health Policy Responses to Epidemiological Change. Vol. 81. No. 1. 15-22.
- McMichael, T. and R. Beaglehole. 2004. The global context for public health. In: Global Public Health: a new era. R. Beaglehole, ed. Oxford, Oxford University Press. 1-23.
- Wilson, R.N. 1970. The Sociology of Health: An Introduction. Random House, New York. 57-68.
- McGavran, E.G. 1958. "The Scientific Diagnosis and Treatment of the Community of the Patient," Public Health News, 38 (Feb. 1958), 61-68.
- United Nations, Food and Agriculture Organization. 2003. Africa and Asia team up to fight AIDS through agriculture. www.fao.org/english/newsroom/field/2003/0303aidsconf.htm
- Sein, T., and U.M. Rafei. 2005. The history and development of public health in developing countries. In: Oxford Textbook of Public Health, Fourth Edition. R. Detels, J. McEwen, R. Beaglehole, and H. Tanaka, eds. 39-61. Oxford: Oxford University Press.
- World Health Organization (WHO). 1999. Nutrition for health and development: progress and prospects on the eve of the twenty-first century. Document WHO/NHD/99.9. WHO, Geneva.
- Scrimshaw, N.S. 1986. Nutrition and Preventive Medicine. In: Maxcy-Rosenau Public health and Preventive medicine, 12th ed., ed. J.M. Last. 1515-1542, Norwalk, CT., Appleton-Century-Crofts.
- Centers for Disease Control and Prevention. 1993. Recommendations of the International Task Force for Disease Eradication. Morbidity and Mortality Weekly Report (MMWR), 42 (RR-16): 1-38.

Don A. Franco

- Miller, M., S. Barrett, and D.A. Henderson. 2006. Control and Eradication. In: Disease Control Priorities in Developing Countries. 2nd Edition. D.T. Jamison, J.G. Breman, A.R. Mearsham, G. Alleyne, M. Claeson, D.B. Evans, P. Jha, A. Miller, and P. Musgrave. Eds. 1163-1176. The International Bank for Reconstruction and Development/The World Bank, Washington, D.C.

- Centers for Disease Control and Prevention. 2001. Morbidity and Mortality Weekly Report (MMWR). International Task Force for Disease Eradication. http://iier.isciii.es/mmwr/preview/mmwrhtml/00001590.htm

- Fenner, F., D.A. Anderson, I. Arita, Z. Jezek, and I.D. Ladnyi. 1988. Smallpox and its eradication. Geneva. World Health Organization.

- Spencer, H.C.: 1991. Dracunculiasis. In: Hunter's Tropical Medicine. G.T. Strickland, ed. 750-756. Philadelphia: W.B. Saunders Co.

- Centers for Disease Control and Prevention. Division of Parasitic Diseases. Fact Sheet. Dracunculiasis. ww.cdc.gov/NCIDOD/DPD/parasites/ dracunculiasis/factsht_dracunculiasis.htm

- www.cwru.edu/med/epidbio/mphp439/Malaria.htm

- Duke, B.O.L.: 1989. Onchocerciasis-river blindness: can it be eradicated? Presented at the Symposium of the International Task Force for Disease Eradication, Atlanta, April 13-14, 1989.

- Benbehani, K.: 1998. Candidate parasitic diseases. In: Global Disease Elimination and Eradication as Public Health Strategies. Proceedings of a Conference held in Atlanta, Georgia, February 23-25, 1998. R.A. Goodman, K.L. Foster, F.L. Trowbridge, and J.P. Figueroa, eds. 64-67. Geneva: World Health Organization.

- Cohen, M.L.: 1998. Candidate bacterial diseases. In: Global Disease Elimination and Eradication as Public Health Strategies. Proceedings of a Conference held in Atlanta, Georgia, February 23-25, 1998. R.A. Goodman, K.L. Foster, F.L. Trowbridge, and J.P. Figueroa, eds. 61-63. Geneva: World Health Organization.

- Hull, H.F., C. de Quadros, J. Bilous et al. 1998. Perspectives from the global poliomyelitis eradication initiative. Proceedings of a Conference held in Atlanta, Georgia, February 23-25, 1998. R.A. Goodman, K.L. Foster, F.L. Trowbridge, and J.P. Figueroa, eds. 42-46. Geneva: WHO.
- www.who.int/infectious-disease-report/pages/ch2text.html
- World Health Organization. 1996. The State of World Health. In the World Health Report 1996 – Fighting disease, fostering development, 1-62. Geneva. World Health Organization.
- Breman, J.G., 1991. Viral Infections with Cutaneous Lesions – Measles. In: Hunter's Tropical Diseases. G.T. Strickland. Ed. 162-166. Philadelphia: W.B. Saunders Co.
- http://ads.emedtv.com/www/delivery/ck.php/oaparams+2 _barnerid+67_zoneid+3_source+www.emedtv.compercent2Finfect ious_disease_cb+faa3fdgcle_maxdest
- Hecht, R., and R. Shah. 2006. Recent Trends and Innovations in Development Assessment for Health. In: Disease Control Priorities in Developing Countries. 2nd Edition. D.T. Jamison, J.G. Breman, A.R. Mearsham, G. Alleyne, M. Claeson, D.B. Evans, P. Jha, A. Miller, and P. Musgrove. Eds. 243-257. The International Bank for Reconstruction and Development/The World bank, Washington, D.C.
- Michaud, C. 2003. Development Assistance for Health: Recent Trends and Resource Allocation. Boston: Harvard Center for Population Development.
- Beaglehole, R. and R. Bonita. 2004. Public Health at the Crossroads, Achievements and Prospects. Second Edition, 227-249. Cambridge University Press, Cambridge.

Chapter 10

- Franco, D.A. 2007. Poverty ~Malnutrition~Disease~Hopelessness: A Cry for Social Justice. Sierra Publishing, Camino, CA.
- Harvard School of Public Health. 2006. HSPH Report: China and India. What's Behind Asia's Gold Rush? Harvard Public Health Review. Summer/Fall 2006. 8-11.

• Hu, H., and N.H. Kim. 1993. Drinking Water Pollution and Human Health. In: Critical Condition: Human Health and the Environment, eds. E. Chivan, A. Haines, H. Hu, and M.McCally. 31-48. Cambridge: Massachusetts Institute of Technology Press.

• Mukherjee, J.S.., and P.E. Farmer. 2006. Infectious Diseases. In: Social Injustice and Public Health, eds. B.S. Levy and V.W. Sidel, 220-237. New York. Oxford University Press.

• Brown, J.L. 2006. Nutrition. In: Social Injustice and Public Health, eds. B.S. Levy and V.W. Sidel, 238-252. New York: Oxford University Press.

• Plough, A. 2006. Promoting Social Justice through Public Health Policies, Programs, and Services. In: Social Injustice and Health. Eds. B.S. Levy and V.W. Sidel. 418-432. New York: Oxford University Press.

• Center for Economic and Social Justice. 1994. Curing World Poverty: The New Role of Property. www.cesj/publications/curingworldpoverty/summary-cwp.htm

Epilogue

• Badgley, R.: 1992. Public Health: Trends and Challenges. In: The crisis of Public Health: Reflections for the Debate, 53-67. The Pan American Health Organization, Scientific Publication 540.

• Powles, J.: 1992. Changes in disease patterns and related social trends. Soc. Sci. Med. 35: 377-387.

• Minkler, M.: 2003. Poverty kills. http://parkridgecenter.org.Page78.html

• http://en.wikipedia.org/wiki/2010 Haitiearthquake

• http://news.yahoo.com/s/ap/cb_haiti_disease_outbreak

• Franco, D.A. 2009. Poverty and the Continuing Global Health Crisis. Tate Publishing Company, Mustang, OK.

About the Author

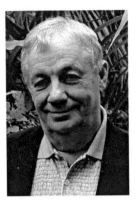

Dr. Don A. Franco has degrees in agriculture, veterinary medicine and public health, and is board certified by the American College of Veterinary Preventive Medicine. He was also made an Honorary Fellow of the Philippine College of Veterinary Public Health for his contributions to the specialty of public health. Dr. Franco is an ardent advocate of the One Medicine-One Health concept, convinced that the future success of the broad and challenging world of medicine necessitates the continuing awareness of the distinct interrelatedness between veterinary medicine and human medicine in the demanding quest for the prevention and control of human diseases, and especially those linked to the animal kingdom that have emerged as significant threats to global health in the past two decades.

Dr. Franco has had adjunct faculty appointments for the past 30 years at both veterinary and medical institutions, and has published extensively in the field of food safety and public health microbiology, including reference texts on food animal and poultry pathology, and several chapters in books on different aspects of food safety, public health microbiology, and the prion diseases.

He has authored three books on poverty and health – *Poverty ~ Malnutrition ~ Disease ~ and Hopelessness: A Cry for Social Justice* (Sierra Publishing, Camino, California), *Poverty and the Continuing Global Health Crisis* (Tate Publishing, Mustang, Oklahoma), and this, his current –*Poverty, Hunger, Disease and Global Health.*

Dr. Franco serves as a public health consultant to the Jerome Foundation of Los Angeles, California, in this foundation's continuing objectives to bring corrective surgery, public health medicine, and educational opportunities to the needy in designated areas of the Philippines. One of the Foundation's outreach programs includes the provision of medical scholarships to worthy students who will after graduation work in regions of the country to help provide health services to the poor, including the RTRMF College of Medicine, Tacloban City, Leyte, where he serves as a Visiting Professor in the Department of Preventive and Community Medicine.

CPSIA information can be obtained at www.ICGtesting.com
Printed in the USA
242687LV00003B/4/P